Day Surgery

96

96

16

D0317381

The book is dedicated to my mother, Janet Oldham, who died before its completion.

D. H.

For Churchill Livingstone:

Commissioning editor: Alex Mathieson
Project manager: Ewan Halley
Project editor: Mairi McCubbin
Project controller: Derek Robertson
Design direction: Judith Wright

Day Surgery
A Nursing Approach

Edited by

Debbie Hodge RGN BSc RCNT DipN PGDE RNT

Principal Lecturer, Department of Post-registration Nursing,
School of Health and Human Sciences,
University of Hertfordshire, Hatfield

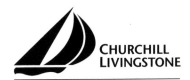
CHURCHILL
LIVINGSTONE

EDINBURGH LONDON NEW YORK PHILADELPHIA SYDNEY TORONTO 1999

CHURCHILL LIVINGSTONE
An Imprint of Harcourt Brace and Company Limited
Churchill Livingstone, Robert Stevenson House, 1–3 Baxter's Place,
Leith Walk, Edinburgh EH1 3AF, UK

First published 1999

ISBN 0 443 05343 X

British Library Cataloguing in Publication Data
A catalogue record for this book is available from the British Library.

Library of Congress Cataloging in Publication Data
A catalog record for this book is available from the Library of Congress.

Medical knowledge is constantly changing. As new information becomes
available, changes in treatment, procedures, equipment and the use of
drugs become necessary. The editor, contributors and the publishers
have, as far as it is possible, taken care to ensure that the information
given in this text is accurate and up to date. However, readers are
strongly advised to confirm that information, especially with regard to
drug usage, complies with the latest legislation and standards of practice.

The authors and publishers have made every effort to trace the copyright
holders for borrowed material. If they have inadvertently over-looked
any, they will be pleased to make the necessary arrangements at the first
opportunity.

The
publisher's
policy is to use
**paper manufactured
from sustainable forests**

Printed in China
NPCC/01

Contents

Contributors

Jill Barker MBBS FRCA MD
Consultant Anaesthetist, Barnet General Hospital, Barnet

5. Pharmacological advances

Maggie Fearon BSc SRN
Wellhouse NHS Trust, Barnet General Hospital, Barnet

10. Quality assurance

Kathryn Rachel Fysh BSc(Hons) RGN
Recovery Co-ordinator, Princess Royal Hospital, Telford

1. Patient selection

Louise Gamble BSc(Hons) RGN RCNT RNT
Joint Programme Leader, Post-registration Bachelor of Nursing,
University of Dundee, Fife Campus, Kirkcaldy

9. Research and day surgery practice

Sarah Grenside BA(Hons) RGN
Senior Lecturer, School of Health and Human Sciences,
University of Hertfordshire, Hatfield

4. Part B Endoscopic or laser procedures undertaken in day surgery

Debbie Hodge RGN BSc RCNT DipN PGDE RNT
Principal Lecturer, Department of Post-registration Nursing,
School of Health and Human Sciences, University of Hertfordshire,
Hatfield

7. Framework for care in day surgery
14. Day surgery as an educational environment

Anna-Marie Kennedy RGN
Sister, The Royal Free Hampstead NHS Trust, London

6. Care of children

Eileen Lock BA(Hons) RN
Day Care Unit Manager, Northwick Park Hospital, Harrow

2. Preparation for procedures

Ian Peate BEd(Hons) MA(Lond)
Senior Lecturer, Department of Adult Nursing and Health Care,
University of Hertfordshire, Hatfield

8. Professional considerations

Bernadette Phelan BSc(Hons) DipN RGN
Clinical Nurse Specialist, Barnet General Hospital, Barnet

4. Part A Common surgical procedures undertaken in day surgery

Jill Solly RGN DMS
Service Manager, Surgery, King's Health Care NHS Trust,
King's College Hospital, London

11. Management in day surgery

Eve Unerman BSc(Hons) RGN DPSN CertEd
Senior Lecturer, School of Health and Human Sciences,
University of Hertfordshire, Barnet

3. Operating room practice

Preface

This book is intended to assist nurses working in a day surgery setting, whether established day surgery nurses or students visiting, working and training in day surgery.

The content follows the day surgery process from assessment, preparation, specific surgical procedures and recovery to discharge home. Specific information on patient selection, preparation and education, and the intervention required for different procedures, is included. A key factor in effective day surgery care is the anaesthetic phase, and a chapter on this particular aspect is also included. Care has been taken in the presentation of the information to make it accessible, with helpful key notes placed in the margins and extensive referencing and further reading provided.

The concept of multi-skilling is emphasised, promoting the day surgery nurse as an expert practitioner. Multi-skilling in this area of practice enables care to be continuous; the same nurse can care for the patient during all aspects of the process.

Chapters on professional issues, research and education are included to help day surgery nurses maintain, develop and extend their professional roles. No day surgery unit, be it free-standing, integrated or ward based, can function without effective leadership, management and quality assurance mechanisms – these essential aspects, along with care planning, are addressed and linked to practical situations.

A project of this kind takes a great deal of energy from a large number of people. I am indebted to all the contributors for sharing their knowledge and practice and I would like to acknowledge the input of Mary Greenos who contributed material on hernia repair, varicose vein surgery, D & C, and hysteroscopy to Chapter 4. Thanks are also due to the day surgery course students at the University of Hertfordshire. They were responsible, in part, for the original idea for the book and in the development of content and practice. In the early stages of the book much work was done in transcribing the content; for this my sincere thanks go to Su Cousins. I am also indebted to my husband Michael and my children, Victoria, Christopher and Stephen, for putting up with a wife and mum who was always talking day surgery! Thanks to all the staff and patients in many day surgery units who have given me the opportunity to both learn and teach in a very exciting area of nursing practice.

Day surgery is now the accepted method of surgical care for a wide variety and increasing number of patients. In order to maintain knowledge and skills I recommend this book to any nurse working in a day surgery environment. May the quality of patient care be enhanced and the professional role for nurses in this speciality continue to develop.

Hertfordshire, 1998   Debbie Hodge

Introduction

The aim of this book is to introduce nurses – those new to day surgery and those who have experience of working in the area – to relevant information related to the journey the patient undertakes in having an operation or procedure as a day case.

Day surgery has had a major impact on both staff and patients. It must be remembered that day surgery is not a new concept. Professor James Nicoll was caring for children on a day basis in the early 1900s and reported his work in Belfast in 1909 (Nicoll 1909). More recently, advances in surgical techniques and pharmacology have led to the expansion of day surgery. Expert surgical intervention for a wide range of procedures can now be provided in a short space of time. For example, a hernia repair in the past may have necessitated a stay in hospital of 7 days; this can now be treated in the day surgery unit in 7 hours (or less in some centres).

Developments in anaesthetic techniques and in new anaesthetic and analgesic drugs allow more patients to be treated on a day basis. Traditionally, only patients from ASA I (see Box 1.1) were considered suitable for day surgery, but with the new developments patients from ASA II and ASA III may now be treated on a day basis. Examples of anaesthetic developments include:

- development and use of propofol, giving an excellent recovery profile with minimal hangover, for use in total intravenous anaesthesia (Millan and Jewkes 1988) and in patient-controlled sedation (Rudkin et al 1992);
- development use of the laryngeal mask, viewed as a valuable tool in anaesthetic practice for day surgery (Pollard & Cooper 1995) although some reservations for certain operations were noted, e.g. tonsillectomy and dental surgery;
- development and use of analgesic and antiemetic drugs, e.g. Alfentanil, Tramadol, non-steroidal antiinflammatory analgesics, Droperidol and Odansetron;
- recognition and use of alternative therapy in day surgery care, e.g. the use of wrist bands providing pressure (acupuncture) at P6 (pericardium 6) point on the flexor surface of the wrist to help with nausea.

Examples of surgical developments include:

- advent of minimally invasive surgery;
- use of laser technology.

Within the UK at the beginning of the 1990s, about 20% of all surgery was performed on a day basis. In 1994, for some procedures (e.g. STOP), the figure was in excess of 60%, and Roberts (1994) noted in his work on accreditation of ambulatory surgery centres that 50% of the most common surgical procedures could be performed on a day basis. In 1993, 50% of elective surgery in North America was performed on a non-inpatient basis, and the figure is projected to increase to 60% (Twersky 1993). These figures have been increasing in recent years, with some centres identifying up to 90% of certain procedures being undertaken on a day basis. However, it must be remembered that demographic and social factors will have a significant part to play in the number of cases of specific procedures that are suitable (or undertaken) as day surgery. Further, while it may be surgically feasible for up to even 100% of instances of a specific operation to be performed as day cases there will always be some patients for whom, for social or medical reasons, day basis care will be unsuitable.

The benefits of ambulatory or day surgery have been well documented (Ghosh 1994). For the patient, these include:

- accurate forward planning, with the operation taking place on the scheduled day and at the scheduled time;
- less time away from home;
- less time off work;
- shorter recovery period.

For the service operators, benefits include:

- fast throughput of patients, making more effective use of operating time;
- easing of pressure on some specialities and reduction in waiting lists;
- maintainance of high quality of care;
- savings in patient hotel costs;
- reduction of out of hours working.

To meet the increasing demands of an expanding day surgery service the concept of the multiskilled practitioner has emerged. This practitioner has knowledge and skill in all of the day surgery processes, from pre-admission assessment through to discharge and follow-up, and contributes to the management and audit of the service.

Specialist courses are now available for nurses working in a day surgery setting, providing an opportunity to develop the multiskilled role. Through expansion and development of these programmes, nurses are developing day surgery into a recognized specialist area of practice, at the forefront of surgical nursing care.

The information in this book is presented in terms of the patient's progression through the day surgery unit, beginning with patient selection and assessment and concluding with such issues as management, research and education. Also included are details and information related to procedures undertaken in a day surgery unit, the nursing framework for care and documentation, care of children, and professional considerations. It is offered as a contribution to the enhancement of practice and to the support of the multiskilled practitioner in day surgery nursing care.

D. H.

REFERENCES

ASA 1991 ASA classification of surgical patients. American Society of Anesthesiology, Chicago.

Ghosh S 1994 Are the Audit Commission's day surgery targets realistic? Journal of One Day Surgery (Autumn): 19–20

Millan J M, Jewkes C F 1988 Recovery and morbidity after day care anaesthesia. Anaesthesiology 4(3): 738

Nicoll J H 1909 The surgery of infancy. British Medical Journal 11: 753–756

Pollard R C, Cooper G M 1995 The laryngeal mask in day surgery: a survey of practice and usage. Ambulatory Surgery 3(i): 37–42

Roberts L 1994 Accreditation of ambulatory surgery centres. Ambulatory Surgery 2(4): 223–226

Rudkin G E et al 1992 Intra-operative patient controlled sedation. Anaesthesia 4(7): 376–381

Twersky R S 1993 To be an out-patient or not to be – selecting the right patients for ambulatory surgery. Ambulatory Surgery 1(1): 5–14

Patient selection

1

Rachel Fysh

■ **CONTENTS**

OVERVIEW

This chapter discusses the factors relating to patient selection and provides examples of assessment criteria.

To determine the suitability of a patient for day surgery, a process of patient selection must take place. Each day surgery unit, following collaboration with surgeons and anaesthetists, will develop guidelines for selection, including nurse assessment, which must be reviewed regularly in order to remain effective in a rapidly changing environment.

It is difficult to make definitive statements about selection, as each unit will develop its own criteria according to surgeons' and anaesthetists' preferences and procedures undertaken, along with the day surgery unit's specific requirements. There can be variations in certain criteria and, although selection has had an impact on cancellation and DNA (did not attend) rates, it is problematic to say whether one set of criteria is superior to another, each having its own merits. Each unit should have guidelines on which to base an informed decision regarding patient suitability, the desired outcomes being that the patient undergoes surgery safely, that patient satisfaction is high, and that maximum utilization of the day surgery unit is achieved.

Whatever selection criteria are used, it is essential that all key personnel are in agreement, to avoid inappropriate selection (as recommended by the Audit Commission 1992). The Audit Commission suggested that the way forward in selecting patients for day surgery should be to consider, as the first step, that all patients are candidates for day surgery. The assessment of patient suitability should then follow. Admission as an inpatient, therefore, should only occur if there are specific medical or social reasons. It is essential that nurses are familiar with and adept at patient assessment. Patient assessment prior to admission for elective surgery in other fields has been reported to show a reduction in cancellations on the day of surgery (Bond 1994, Nelson 1995).

PROCEDURE SUITABILITY

Patient selection may begin in the outpatient clinic, with the initial decision being made by the clinician, or in the GP's surgery where diagnosis and indication for surgery are defined. As developments progress, and patients meet specific anaesthetic criteria, referral to the day surgery unit for surgery may come directly from the GP's surgery (Bradshaw et al 1994).

The selection process begins by establishing whether the procedure is suitable for day surgery. This decision may vary between day surgery units and is continuously revised as surgical techniques and anaesthesia develop. In general terms, acceptable procedures will meet the following criteria:

- The procedure should not exceed 60 minutes.
- The procedure is unlikely to cause pain and discomfort that would necessitate injected analgesia after discharge.
- The procedure should not require drains or specialized nursing care.
- Postoperative bleeding is unlikely.

PATIENT ASSESSMENT

When the decision has been made that the procedure is appropriate for day surgery, the process of patient assessment takes place. This process is vital to ensure patient safety and the efficient use of the day surgery unit.

Guidelines for selection are required to take into account physiological, sociological and psychological factors that affect the process and its outcome. Following the initial referral for day surgery, an assessment is carried out, usually by an assessment nurse.

Where assessments have been delegated to nurses, the 1992 Audit Commission reports, positive feedback is obtained. The identification, at this stage, of unsuitable patients for day surgery is necessary to reduce the number of patients being cancelled on the day of surgery – thus, reports Lloyd et al (1994), improving day surgery utilization and the safety and convenience of patients. The report of the Task Force set up by the UK National Health Service Management Executive (1993) states that inappropriate selection of patients will adversely affect the quality of outcome for both the patients and the unit.

Physiological parameters

Medical conditions

It has been standard practice that only patients who fulfil the standards set by the American Society of Anesthesiologists' classification of physical status ASA I or ASA II (see Box 1.1) are suitable for day surgery anaesthesia. Some units, however, may consider patients in ASA physical status Class III whose systemic disease is well controlled. There are obvious implications of increased admission rates and occurrence of complications that could prevent the smooth running of the theatre list and result in additional anaesthetic and nursing time associated with this group of patients. A degree of flexibility may result in inappropriate selection and, for this

■ **BOX 1.1 The American Society of Anesthesiologists' (ASA) classification of physical status (reproduced with permission from the Royal College of Surgeons, England, 1992)**

Class I: Patient has no organic, physiological, biochemical or psychiatric disturbance. The pathological process for which surgery is to be performed is localized and does not entail a systemic disturbance. *Examples*: a fit patient with an inguinal hernia; a fibroid uterus in an otherwise healthy woman.

Class II: Mild to moderate systemic disturbance caused either by the condition to be treated surgically or by other pathophysiological processes. *Examples*: slightly limiting organic heart disease; mild diabetes; essential hypertension or anaemia.

Class III: Severe systemic disturbance or disease from whatever cause, even though it may not be possible to define the degree of disability with finality. *Examples*: severely limiting organic heart disease; severe diabetes with vascular complications; moderate to severe degrees of pulmonary insufficiency; angina pectoris, or healed myocardial infarction.

Class IV: Severe systemic disorders that are already life threatening, not always correctable by operation. *Examples*: patients with organic heart disease showing marked signs of cardiac insufficiency; persistent angina, or active myocarditis; advanced degrees of pulmonary, hepatic, renal, or endocrine insufficiency.

Class V: The moribund patient who has little chance of survival but is submitted to operation in desperation. *Examples:* burst abdominal aneurysm with profound shock; major cerebral trauma with rapidly increasing intracranial pressure; massive pulmonary embolus. Most of these patients require operation as a resuscitative measure with little, if any, anaesthesia.

reason, if these patients are selected initially from outpatients, the consultant anaesthetist must be consulted prior to the patient's being accepted.

The following medical conditions may contraindicate day surgery:

1. diabetes – unless well controlled by diet alone;
2. cardiac disease – any apparent overt cardiac disease, including the following:
   - angina
   - heart murmur
   - pacemaker
   - MI within the last 2 years;
3. hypertension:
   - BP > 160/100 if 60 years or under,
   - >180/100 if aged over 60 years;

4. respiratory disease – any chronic respiratory disease; asthma is usually acceptable if controlled, chest clear and attacks have not resulted in hospital admission;
5. arthritis – severe limiting arthritis, especially of neck, jaw or hands;
6. neurological or muscular disorders – significant neurological or muscular disease; epilepsy with any episode of fit in the past year or after previous anaesthetic;
7. blood disorders – bleeding tendency, anaemia, sickle cell anaemia;
8. pregnancy – unless in agreement with obstetrician and anaesthetist;
9. hepatitis B and HIV – infected or potentially infected;
10. micturition – patients liable to postoperative retention of urine;
11. medication – patients currently taking the following:
    - steroids
    - MAOIs
    - hypoglycaemic drugs
    - clonidine
    - glyceryl trinitrate
    - aminophylline
    - digoxin
    - anticoagulants
    - oral contraceptives – in the 6 weeks prior to leg operations.

Further physiological assessment of patients need to take into account age, weight, and results of appropriate investigations.

Age

The Royal College of Surgeons (1992) suggested that the upper age limit is in the range 65–70 years. This is dependent on a number of factors; a patient aged 75 years presenting as fit and healthy, without medical or social contraindications, may be more suitable than a younger patient with a complex medical history. Studies have demonstrated that an arbitrary age limit for patients who are physical status I or II is unwarranted (Meridy 1982). When considering age it is worth remembering, however, that the elderly may have other problems relating to the aging process that may make day surgery non-viable.

The lower age limit is less well defined, with some day surgery units setting this at 1 year of age, while others accept younger patients. Essentially, the lower age limit is dependent on the facilities of the unit and is also governed by the operational policy of each unit. Ideally there should be separate areas for children which can accommodate children, parents and a play area. Further considerations to care of children are given in Chapter 6.

Weight

Obesity is a major consideration in day surgery, presenting technical difficulties for the anaesthetist, surgeon and nursing staff during anaesthetic administration, surgery and recovery. Obese patients are also susceptible to other medical conditions, e.g. hypertension, and there is an increased risk of complications; therefore, obese patients are generally excluded for day surgery. In determining an acceptable limit, it may be necessary to consider the type of surgery being performed. In laparoscopy an upper weight limit of 80 kg has been suggested by Carrington (1993), because of the difficulties encountered in performing this type of surgery on larger patients. However, if 80 kg were used as a more general criterion it would exclude many people who would otherwise be suitable. The weight of a patient alone is not an ideal method of measuring obesity – height should also be taken into consideration. The Body Mass Index (BMI) takes account of weight and height and is a more suitable indicator of obesity, with day surgery units setting an upper BMI limit. This is variable but the upper limit is commonly between 30 and 33, as is shown in Figure 1.1. Patients who are rejected because of weight problems may request help and advice.

Investigations

Investigations start with the taking of baseline observations – pulse rate, blood pressure and urinalysis – which may themselves highlight a problem: e.g. hypertension, which would require treatment and stabilization before the patient could be considered for surgery. Following the taking of a patient's history, it may become evident that further investigations are required before the patient's suitability can be confirmed.

The taking of routine investigations have major cost implications for a day surgery unit and result in an increased demand on the resources of haematology, ECG and X-ray departments. Any investigation once ordered must be retrieved and examined and demands the time not only of the assessment nurse but also that of the anaesthetist.

It is important to remember that any investigation may result in a patient's being cancelled. Assessment, therefore, must occur within an acceptable time-frame for the tests to be retrieved and checked. The assessment nurse must ensure that *all* tests have been carried out prior to surgery and care must be taken to safeguard that *all* test results have

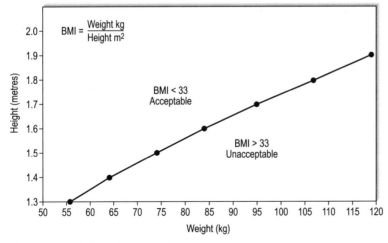

Figure 1.1 Body Mass Index (BMI).

been checked thoroughly. As Merli et al (1993) point out, *ignoring or not observing abnormal results of routine investigations creates added legal risk.* However, Fisher & Krzeminska (1994) reported that there appeared to be little evidence to support routine testing of patients and suggested that investigations be carried out only on the basis of history, examination and assessment. Performing investigations on these criteria depends on clinical judgement. This may not be appropriate for day surgery units who do not have personnel skilled in patient assessment.

> Where routine investigations have been ordered, these must be followed up, as ignoring or not observing abnormal results creates added legal risk.

If routine investigations are adopted, then the following are appropriate for day surgery patients undergoing general anaesthesia:

- haemoglobin – required for all females (after puberty); males over 50 years of age; history of anaemia or clinically anaemic;
- urea, electrolytes – required for all patients aged over 50 years; under 50 years if diuretics, antihypertensive or cardiac drugs are being taken; kidney or urinary problems, other than the reason for admission;
- blood glucose – glycosuria or suspected diabetes or hypoglycaemia;
- chest X-ray – acute respiratory symptoms; possible metastases; suspected or established cardiorespiratory disease with no chest X-ray in last 12 months;
- ECG – all patients over 50 years and any patient suspected of cardiac disease (if no ECG in last 3 months);
- clotting screen / platelet count – known or suspected liver disease; very high alcohol intake; personal/family history of abnormal bleeding;
- sickledex – patients of Afro-Caribbean origin and the result of a previous sickle cell test unknown;
- hepatitis B screen – history of jaundice not due to gallstones or infectious hepatitis;
- beta HCG – if pregnancy suspected; immediately prior to laparoscopic sterilization;
- group and save – termination of pregnancy.

Psychological parameters

Patients selected for day surgery may be uncertain of what lies ahead and may, as a result of a rushed outpatients appointment, present to assessment with many questions and concerns unanswered. In order to reduce anxiety, the assessment must allow enough time to answer patients' questions, ensuring that they understand and are happy with the reply. Patients may well come with preconceived ideas about day surgery, which may be causing them concern, in addition to the anxiety of undergoing surgery. Research has documented (Boore 1978, Haywood 1975) the value of preoperative preparation in reducing anxiety and pain. These two factors can be responsible for delayed recovery and could result in overnight admission.

For an assessment, adequate time must be allocated to allow the patient to discuss planned care and discharge procedure; verbal information should be fully supported by written information. This information must be relevant and accurate if it is to be effective. The Task Force (1993) set up by the NHS reported that lack of information was a problem area.

Time taken during assessment to explain, answer questions and educate the patient will result in improved patient preparation.

Part of the education process involves explaining to the patient what to expect on the day of surgery, the procedure itself, and what to expect during recovery and at discharge on returning home. Armed with this information, the patient can make an informed decision regarding their proposed visit for surgery and what arrangements are required regarding work and family.

A thorough assessment might reveal patients for whom the prospect of day surgery is just too much for them to comprehend. These patients might best be suited for inpatient admission and should be referred.

Day surgery requires the patient to adhere to specific pre- and postoperative instructions, and for this reason the patient's ability to understand and comply with these is essential. If there is doubt about a patient's ability, then the patient must be referred for inpatient surgery to ensure their safety and to minimize potential postoperative problems.

Social parameters

Day surgery demands suitable home circumstances and ongoing care from responsible carers. There is no justification for discharging a patient to the care of someone who is unable to fulfil the role of carer due to ill health or infirmity, or to unsuitable home conditions. For this reason it is essential that at assessment the social criteria are addressed to ensure safety on returning home. Key aspects are:

> It is essential to address social criteria to ensure safety of the patient on returning home.

- a responsible and physically able adult to look after them for 24–36 hours after the operation;
- an escort to drive them home by private car or to accompany them in a taxi;
- access to a telephone (either at home or close by);
- easy access to the home, or place of care, with an indoor toilet;
- residence no more than a one-hour journey from the hospital.

If patients have not been made aware of these criteria prior to surgery, it may result in overnight admission purely for social reasons. A fully informed patient is best placed to ensure that the social criteria are met. It has been noted, however, that in some instances patients have actually driven themselves home even though advised to the contrary (Markanday & Platzer 1994). Therefore it may be advisable for patients to confirm in writing that they understand that there may be prolonged effects from anaesthetics and, therefore, they should not drive, operate machinery, or sign important documents for 48 hours postoperatively. Most patients, if advised in advance, will be able to meet these requirements, but for others it may not be practical. These patients can be accommodated in a Hospital Hotel, if available, or will be referred for inpatient admission.

Nursing assessment of patients

Assessment of patients is invaluable in identifying patients 'at risk' and in reducing cancellations, DNA (did not attend) rates, and unplanned admissions, as reported by the 1992 Audit Commission. The reduction of these areas resulted in improved utilization of the day surgery unit, theatre time and, ultimately, reduced waiting lists – thus benefitting all patients.

The creation of the role of the assessment nurse in day surgery has resulted from the identification of a need for accurate and thorough assessment, a need for accurate patient information and education, and careful discharge planning. Clinicians in a busy outpatient department are not best placed for such a thorough assessment, and patients often find themselves with a list of questions unanswered. The 1992 Audit Commission suggested that units where this role has been developed have seen improvements in the service with regard to decreased DNA rates and fewer problems on the day of procedure.

The question arises as to where and when preadmission assessment should be undertaken. It may be possible for the patient to be assessed in the outpatient department by a nurse from the day surgery unit, or to attend the day surgery unit directly after an outpatient appointment. Alternatively, perhaps specific preadmission assessment clinics may be set up. Each approach has its own particular merits and disadvantages, as will be noted later.

The necessary skills required of an assessment nurse involve:

- the ability to communicate at all levels;
- the ability to provide accurate information and have in-depth knowledge of procedures and day surgery requirements;
- the ability to assess, plan and evaluate;
- the ability to make decisions;
- the ability to review and improve the service.

In addition, the ability to provide an accurate assessment of suitability for day surgery, along with an overview of the whole experience – from selection, surgery, to recovery and discharge – is vital if the patient is to understand and participate in his own care and so promote the best possible outcome.

The Patient's Charter has brought to the fore the patient's right to be given a clear explanation of any treatment proposed. This is further supported by the report of the Task Force (1993) that recommended briefing patients in advance as best practice.

The aims of assessment are shown in Box 1.2, and can be met by the assessment nurse by applying the identified skills. To undertake this, the nurse must be prepared through appropriate educational and experiential programmes.

Specific day surgery courses are now available, and investment in the training of assessment nurses can only be seen as a positive move towards improved patient care and day surgery utilization. The need for such training has been recognized (Task Force 1993), and this must not be ignored if nurses are to make significant contributions to day surgery.

In determining a suitable candidate for a nurse-led assessment clinic, the skills required need to be considered, and the decision to rotate staff needs to be taken. The advantage of having flexible nursing staff with the ability to rotate and perform competently in all areas of day surgery has

> ■ **BOX 1.2 The aims of assessment**
>
> - to provide information – oral and written;
> - to alleviate anxiety;
> - to educate patients and discuss pain management;
> - to confirm patient suitability for day surgery;
> - to perform, and examine, appropriate investigations prior to admission;
> - to refer unsuitable patients for inpatient treatment;
> - to prepare patients for their admission;
> - to prepare patients and their carers for discharge;
> - to reduce administrative documentation on admission;
> - to improve day surgery utilization and theatre time by reducing cancellations, DNAs and unplanned admissions;
> - to increase patient satisfaction.

been highlighted by the NHS Management Executive (1991) as invaluable at times of shortage. Rotation would provide increased knowledge of assessment, operative procedures, patient care and discharge. It could be argued, however, that rotating staff dilutes skills. Giving out poor information has been highlighted as a problem area (Task Force 1993) and it may be advantageous to have a permanent assessment nurse who will become an expert practitioner in this area.

The development of nurse practitioners within the Scope of Professional Practice will see the role of the assessment nurse change. This role may evolve to that of a nurse practitioner, who will be ideally placed to ensure the best possible service for patients.

When considering day surgery patients it is important to remember that what can be seen as a 'minor' procedure by healthcare professionals is probably perceived by the patient as a 'major' experience. The nurse undertaking assessment plays a vital role in preparing patients – not just physically and socially but, of equal importance, psychologically.

There are some disadvantages to attending assessment clinics, however, and alternatives may need to be sought. For example, it may be necessary to assess a patient over the telephone if they are unable to attend a clinic. This practice is far from ideal and may result in a cancellation on the day of surgery. It could be argued that this contact is better than none at all. Even so, it is not possible to accurately assess and plan patient care by this method.

When comparing the advantages of assessment, as seen in Box 1.3, with the disadvantages (Box 1.4), it would appear that the advantages of assessment significantly outweigh the disadvantages.

Assessment of carers

Following a patient's initial recovery in the day surgery unit, the recovery process continues at home with the emphasis of care being placed with the

■ **BOX 1.3 Advantages of assessment**

- Improves unit utilization by reducing cancellations, DNAs and unplanned admissions.
- Allows patients presenting with certain conditions to be treated, thus avoiding cancellation on the day of surgery.
- Provides a relaxed environment where the patient is given the opportunity to ask questions.
- Allows pre- and postoperative instructions to be given at a time when patients are more receptive.
- Reduces anxiety by keeping patients informed and by visiting the unit.
- Allows patients to plan for surgery; this improves/enhances aftercare.
- Allows preoperative investigations to be performed if deemed necessary.
- Reduces nursing administration on admission.
- Increases patient satisfaction.

■ **BOX 1.4 Disadvantages of assessment**

- May require patients to have a separate appointment if preadmission assessment is not appropriate at time of outpatient appointment.
- May result in patients incurring additional travelling expenditure.
- May be inconvenient for some patients because of other commitments.
- May appear inappropriate for those patients who are young, otherwise fit and healthy, and who are already informed.

Patients and carers must be fully informed about what to expect postoperatively and what to do in the event of complications.

carer. *Patients and carers must, therefore, be fully informed about what to expect and what to do in the event of complications.* Some patients may have unrealistic expectations, and it is the responsibility of the day surgery unit to ensure that patients receive appropriate information on what to expect at home and how to manage. This information should be given in advance and not simply on the day of surgery as discharge information. Patients will only be discharged from the day surgery unit when they have met the discharge criteria, which are shown in Figure 1.2. Following discharge some patients may experience nausea, headaches, muscle pains, blurred vision, pain and, possibly, anxiety associated with having had a general anaesthetic. For ill-informed patients and carers these may cause considerable concern. That is why postoperative information must be available to the carer. Carers are also given a contact telephone number in the event of a problem occurring. The time taken to assess a patient's home circumstances and the carer during assessment will be time well spent.

Some procedures will be such that patients will require district nurse support. Each day surgery unit should have a link with a community

Discharge criteria	Yes	No
1 Has stable BP and pulse		
2 Can swallow and cough		
3 Can walk without feeling faint		
4 Has minimal nausea and is not vomiting		
5 Can breathe comfortably and colour is normal		
6 Is wide awake and is aware of what is going on		
7 Has passed urine		
8 Has taken fluids and food		
9 Has had the operation site checked		
10 Has had their postoperative instructions (verbal/written)		
11 Has had their postoperative medication		
12 Has their GP's letter		
13 Has outpatient appointment		
14 Has someone to take them home		
15 Has someone to stay overnight		
16 District nurse arranged		

Figure 1.2 Example of a discharge criteria form.

liaison nurse. For procedures that are known to require this support, the community liaison nurse should be informed at the time of assessment, with confirmation given on the day of surgery. For other patients, they may simply need to visit their GP for removal of sutures. A system for informing patients' GPs must be in operation. It is important to ensure that communication links are established and maintained with GPs and community nurses to keep them fully informed to ensure continuity of care. The Audit Commission (1992) reported that GPs have had only a slight increase in their workload as a result of day surgery. As day surgery develops, however, a greater impact on community services, with more support required for carers, may be seen.

For those patients who do not require district nurse support, the provision of a telephone followup service (on the following day) provides support and reassurance. This allows the opportunity to check on a patient's progress, to reinforce information, and to answer any questions that a patient or carer may have. This service should prevent a rise in the number of patients seeking advice from their GP postoperatively. It may be beneficial for day surgery units to adopt a questionnaire aimed specifically at carers. To date, there is little research in this area of patient care and, as day surgery develops, it is this group that is at the forefront of patient care.

Process, documentation and outcome

In some hospitals the assessment process for day surgery patients will take place in the outpatient clinic. In others it will be carried out by an assessment nurse, usually in the day surgery itself. Where the surgery is scheduled to take place within 4–6 weeks, the patient can be assessed on the same day as the outpatient appointment. However, if the period exceeds 4–6 weeks, or for waiting list patients, it is necessary to recall the patient for assessment. The reason for recalling patients nearer to the date of surgery is that patients' circumstances and medical condition may have changed. Any investigations undertaken may also be invalid. Recalling patients for assessment may be inconvenient for some, but the advantages of assessment far outweigh the disadvantages.

Patients book an appointment with the day surgery unit to attend for assessment. The patient and the assessment nurse go through and complete a questionnaire. The necessity for further investigations will become apparent at this stage according to agreed guidelines. Routine observations of pulse, blood pressure, height, weight and urinalysis will take place at this time. The length of time required for assessment will vary according to an individual's needs, but 20–30 minutes is usually adequate. An example of an assessment form is given in Figure 1.3, and the corresponding guidelines are given in Figure 1.4. Guidelines for appropriate investigations have been mentioned under physiological parameters but, as discussed previously, these will be specifically developed by the anaesthetist involved and according to unit policy.

The assessment form shown is comprehensive and applies for adult patients. When considering the suitability of children for day surgery it is appropriate to adopt a specific paediatric assessment form as shown in Figure 1.5.

Following completion of the assessment form the opportunity exists for answering the patient's questions, providing relevant information and patient education, if applicable. It is during this period that the patient will be most receptive, but oral information must be supported by written material, thus ensuring that patients and carers are fully informed. In cases where patient suitability relies on the results of investigations, then the patient must receive confirmation as soon as possible. Patient assessment may highlight a problem that is reversible, e.g. hypertension. This will require that the patient be postponed, unless postponement would be detrimental, and the patient referred back to the GP. Once resolved, the GP will inform the day surgery unit and the patient's surgery will proceed. Patients who do not meet the criteria for day surgery will be referred for inpatient admission and informed of the reason. These patients may well require a degree of counselling with the assessment nurse, as they are likely to be apprehensive about the reason for being rejected.

Once a patient has been assessed and confirmed as suitable for day surgery, she will be appropriately prepared physically and psychologically on her arrival. Assessing patients beforehand reduces nursing documentation and preparation on the day of surgery; however, it is necessary to complete the immediate preoperative documentation. This includes confirming that

Date.......................   Home Tel. No...........................   Age ....

Contact Personal Tel. No...

Next of kin.....................................   Escort ....

Name of GP...............................   Consultant ....

Address of GP...

Proposed procedure...

| Patient sticker |

Please tick (✓) applicable box below

	Yes	No	Nurse's comments
1 Are you willing to undergo the proposed treatment as a day patient?			

Will you–

	Yes	No	Nurse's comments
2 Be able to be driven home by private car?			
3 Have easy access from transport to your home?			
4 Have someone to take you home?			
5 Have a telephone at home?			
6 Have easy access to a lavatory inside your home?			
7 Have someone at home able to look after you for 36 hours?			

Have you ever suffered from any of the following?

	Yes	No	Nurse's comments
8 Chest pain on exercise or at night			
9 Breathlessness			
10 Asthma or bronchitis			
11 High blood pressure			
12 Heart murmur			
13 Fainting easily			
14 Convulsions or fits			
15 Jaundice (yellowness)			
16 Indigestion or heartburn			
17 Kidney or urinary problem			
18 Anaemia or other blood problems			
19 Deep vein thrombosis or pulmonary embolism			
20 Excessive bleeding or bruising			
21 Arthritis			
22 Muscle disease or progressive weakness			
23 Diabetes			

TCI date ....

Figure 1.3 Example of an assessment form for care in the day unit. Adapted from The Royal College of Surgeons of England (1992).

	Please tick (✓) applicable box below		
Have you ever had–	**Yes**	**No**	**Nurse's comments**
24 A heart attack?			
25 A serious illness, for example, rheumatic fever?			
26 Allergy or reaction to medicines, elastoplast etc?			List allergies below
Do you–			
27 Take any medicines (tablets, patches, injections, inhalers etc)?			List medicines below
Do you–			
28 Smoke?			
29 Drink more than 1½ pints of beer or 3 shorts a day?			
30 Have any reason to suspect you may be a carrier of Hepatitis B virus or HIV (Aids)?			
31 If a woman, are you pregnant or taking the pill?			Name of contraceptive pill
Is there anything else the surgeon/anaesthetist should know?			
Do you have any questions about the procedure?			

34 What operations have you had before, if any
(please list starting with the most recent)?

1. ....

2. ....

3. ....

4. ....

35 Did you have any anaesthetic or surgical
complications (please list)?

1. ....

2. ....

36 When was your most recent anaesthetic?

....

Figure 1.3 (contd)

37 Has any blood relative had a problem with anaesthetics?

Yes ☐   No ☐

38 How long will it take you to travel home?

.... Hours...................... Minutes

39 Do you have any of the following (please circle)?

Dentures   Crowned   Loose   Contact   Hearing   Pacemaker
              teeth   teeth   lenses   aid

I understand that there may be prolonged effects from anaesthetics which make it unsafe for me to drive, operate any form of machinery, drink alcohol or make important decisions for 36 hours after a general anaesthetic, and confirm that the answers I have given above are true to the best of my knowledge.

Parent/guardian signature ....

Further enquiry required   if 'NO' for numbers 1–7
                                or 'YES' for numbers 8–39

Investigations required

Hb	130 – 180 g/l (male)	ECG
	115 – 164 g/l (female)	
		CXR
Sodium	135 – 147 mmol/l	
		Other(list)
Potassium	3.8 – 5.0 mmol/l	
Creatinine	60 – 120 mmol/l	ECG

Nurse observations

Pulse   .... bpm reg/irreg   BP   (1)..........mmHg

Heart   .... bpm (if pulse irreg)   (1)..........mmHg

Weight .... kg   Height.......... cm

Urine   .... Sugar

          .... Protein

Acceptable for day care anaesthesia   YES ☐   NO ☐   **REFER** ☐
                                                         (Anaesthetist,
                                                         surgeon, GP)

Nurse's signature ....

Doctor's signature ....

Figure 1.3 (contd)

1	If not willing	NOT SUITABLE
2	If not possible to arrange transport	NOT SUITABLE
3	If difficult	NOT SUITABLE
4	If not possible to arrange escort	NOT SUITABLE
5	If reasonable access cannot be arranged	NOT SUITABLE
6	Depending on circumstances and procedure	MAY NOT BE SUITABLE
7	If not possible to arrange	NOT SUITABLE
8	If pain occurs at rest	NOT SUITABLE
	If pain occurs when walking on the flat	
	If pain normally well controlled and occurs only in exceptional circumstances request ECG and CXR	
	If abnormal	NOT SUITABLE
9	If breathlessness occurs when walking on the flat	NOT SUITABLE
10	If patient's normal activity is limited	NOT SUITABLE
	If well controlled request CXR and Spirometry	
	If CXR abnormal or FEVi or FVC <70% of predicted	NOT SUITABLE
11	If blood pressure taken regularly and well controlled, take blood pressure	NOT SUITABLE
	If greater than 160/100 mmHg (or more than 180/100 if between 60–70 years) repeat	
	If remains greater	NOT SUITABLE
12	If clear history of heart murmer	NOT SUITABLE
13	Record what causes fainting	
	If on excercise or if patient is over 60 years	NOT SUITABLE
14	If epileptic and well controlled on medication	SUITABLE
	If epileptic fit within last year or with an anaesthetic	NOT SUITABLE
15	If jaundice was due to gall stones or infectious hepatitis	SUITABLE
	If jaundice possible due to hepatitis B request hepatitis B screen	
	If positive	NOT SUITABLE
16	If due to hiatus hernia reliably diagnosed– but consider prescription of H2 antagonist over preoperative night	SUITABLE
	If possible myocardia ischaemia request medical opinion	NOT SUITABLE
17	If the reason for treatment	SUITABLE
	If not the reason for treatment request U & E	
	If abnormal	NOT SUITABLE
	If severe difficulty with micturation	NOT SUITABLE
18	If recently anaemic request FBC	
	If Hb < 10 g/dl adult	
	If Hb < 11 g/dl child	NOT SUITABLE
	If haemophiliac	NOT SUITABLE
	If known to have sickle cell train (or disease)	NOT SUITABLE
	If of Caribbean, East Mediterranean, Middle or Far Eastern origin and result of sickle test unknown request sickle cell test	

Figure 1.4 Guidelines for nurse assessment. Adapted from The Royal College of Surgeons of England (1992).

19	If clear history of DVT or pulmonary embolism	NOT SUITABLE
20	If required hospital treatment	NOT SUITABLE
	Has bleeding been excessive following tooth extraction, or bruising occured without a known cause?	
	If yes request clotting screen	
	If abnormal	NOT SUITABLE
	Is there a family history? If so, or any doubt request clotting screen	
	If abnormal	NOT SUITABLE
21	If the patient is severely disabled	NOT SUITABLE
	If neck involved inform anaesthetist	SUITABLE
22	If normal activity compromised (e.g. multiple sclerosis, motor neurone disease)	NOT SUITABLE
	If the patient has myasthenia gravis	NOT SUITABLE
	If there is a family history of cataracts	NOT SUITABLE
	If there is a history of poliomyelitis which required assisted ventilation or was associated with swallowing difficulties	NOT SUITABLE
	Otherwise, including ME syndrome	SUITABLE
23	If tablet or insulin dependent diabetic	NOT SUITABLE
24	If MI within 2 years	NOT SUITABLE
25	Record list of serious medical illnesses	
26	Record all allergies	
27	Record nature of medication, dose and duration	
	If on steroid or anticoagulation treatment, hypoglycaemics, catapres	NOT SUITABLE
28	Record number of cigarettes/ounces of tobacco smoked	
	Discourage smoking until operation	
29	Record average consumption of alcohol	
	It is recommended that the upper limit for men is 3 units and for women 2 units per day	
	Advise patient of this if above limit	
	If reason to believe abusing alcohol order LFTs	
	If normal	SUITABLE
30	If suspected	NOT SUITABLE
31	Pregnancy : establish that referring clinician is aware of this	
	If not refer back	
	Pill/HRT : Oestrogen-containing pills should be stopped for 6 weeks preoperatively on patients having operations on legs or of long duration	
	NB advise alternative contraception	
32	If concerned inform surgeon or anaesthetist	
33	Try to answer the question(s)	
	If concerned inform the surgeon or anaesthetist	

Figure 1.4 (contd)

Further enquiries for numbers 34–39

34 If you suspect these may affect suitability for day case surgery
    seek a medical opinion

35 Record any serious complications

36 Record when last anaesthetic

37 If a family history of malignant hyperthermia   NOT SUITABLE
    If a family history of scoline or suxamethonium sensitivity
    inform anaesthetist
    If other significant problems or if in doubt as to suitability of day case
    surgery seek medical opinion

38 No more than one hour's journey is desirable

39 Record pacemaker   NOT SUITABLE

**If considered unsuitable for day surgery the patient should
be told the reason and be referred back to the surgeon.
The general practitioner should be informed.**

Figure 1.4 (contd)

data gathered at assessment is still correct. Other documentation will include consent form, anaesthetic form, theatre check list, care plan and discharge protocol.

In conclusion, as day surgery evolves and with more procedures being undertaken, preadmission assessment of patients will play a major role in ensuring an efficient and safe service. A satisfactory outcome relies on patients receiving their surgery safely, with maximum utilization of the day surgery unit. Appropriate patient selection, including assessment, will ensure this outcome.

As preadmission assessment of patients becomes accepted, and as patients from ASA Classes II and III form part of the day surgery population, it may be deemed necessary for the nursing staff to undertake specific investigations, e.g. blood screening and ECG. In doing so, nurses will be expanding their role, but these should only be carried out after the relevant education, supervision and practice.

The expansion of the assessment role may well provide a swifter and more efficient service for patients.

FURTHER READING

Bradshaw C, Pritchett C, Eccles M, Armitage T, Wright H, Todd E 1994 South Tyneside 'fastrack' day surgery planning. Journal of One-day Surgery 3(4): 6
Vijay V, King T, Knowles L 1995 Preliminary experience of a day surgery assessment clinic. Journal of One-day Surgery 4(3): 7–8

REFERENCES

Audit Commission 1992 All in a day's work: an audit of day surgery in England and Wales. NHS occasional papers. HMSO, London

Date................. Preferred name .... Age ....

Next of kin .... Tel. No. ....

Person collecting .... Tel. No. ....

| Patient sticker |

Name of GP..

Address of GP..Consultant ....

Proposed procedure...

Please tick (✓) applicable box below

	Yes	No	Nurse's comments
1 Are you willing for your child to undergo the proposed treatment as a day patient?			
Will this be your child's first operation?			
Has your child got a cough, cold or nose trouble?			
10 Has your child had bronchitis, asthma or other chest trouble?			
12 Has your child had heart disease or rheumatic fever?			
13 Does your child faint easily?			
14 Has your child had convulsions or fits?			
15 Has your child ever been jaundiced?			
17 Has your child ever had urinary or kidney trouble?			
18 Does your child have anaemia or other blood problems?			
20 Does your child bruise or bleed excessively?			
23 Has your child ever had diabetes or sugar in the urine?			
25 Has your child had any serious illnesses?			
26 Does your child have allergies or reactions to medicines etc?			
27 Is your child on any medicines now (tablets, capsules, injections, inhalers etc.)?			
Is your child up to date with immunisations?			
30 Have you any reason to suspect your child may be a carrier of Hepatitis B virus or HIV (Aids)?			
33 Do you have any questions about the procedure?			
36 Has your child any problems with anaesthetics?			
Is there anything else the surgeon/anaesthetist should know?			
39 Has your child any loose teeth at present?			

Admission date ....

Parents please note that after your child's anaesthetic he/she should not ride a bicycle nor play unsupervised for 24 hours following a general anaesthetic

Figure 1.5 Example of paediatric assessment form for care in the day case unit. Adapted from The Royal College of Surgeons of England (1992), with thanks to R. Brazier RGN.

34 What operations has your child had before, if any
(please list starting with the most recent)?

1. ....

2. ....

3. ....

4. ....

35 Did she/he have any anaesthetic or surgical
complications (please list)?

1. ....

2. ....

36 When was her/his most recent anaesthetic?

....

37 Has any blood relative had a problem with anaesthetics?

Yes ☐   No ☐

38 How long will it take you to travel home?

.... Hours .... Minutes

39 Does your child have any of the following (please circle)?

Dentures   Crowned   Loose   Contact   Hearing   Pacemaker
            teeth   teeth   lenses   aid

I understand that after my child's anaesthetic he/she should not ride a bicycle nor play unsupervised
for 24 hours following a general anaesthetic and confirm that the answers I have given above
are true to the best of my knowledge.

Parent/guardian signature ....

Figure 1.5 (contd)

Bond D 1994 Patient assessment before surgery. Clinical Orthopaedics 8(28): 23–28
Boore J 1978 Prescription for recovery. Royal College of Nursing, London
Bradshaw C, Pritchett C, Eccles M, Armitage T, Wright H, Todd E 1994 South Tyneside
    'fastrack' day surgery planning. Journal of One-day Surgery 3(4): 6
Carrington S 1993 Day surgery in Bristol. British Journal of Theatre Nursing
    (February): 12–15
Fisher A, Krzeminska E 1994 Adult day case anaesthesia. In: Day case anaesthesia and
    sedation. Blackwell Scientific, Oxford
Haywood J 1975 Information – a prescription against pain. Royal College of Nursing,
    London
Lloyd S, Clark C, Small D, Donnell L 1994 A patient operated computer system for
    assessing fitness for day surgery anaesthesia. Journal of One-day Surgery 3(4): 3
Markanday L, Platzer H 1994 Brief encounters. Nursing Times 90(7)
Meridy H W 1982 Criteria for selection of ambulatory surgical patients and guidelines for

anaesthetic management – a retrospective study of 1553 cases. Anaesthesia and Analgesia 61(11): 921–926

Merli G J, Weitz H H, Lubin M F 1993 Medical consultation. Medical Clinics of North America 77(2): 289–308

NHS Management Executive 1991 Day surgery: making it happen. Value for money unit. HMSO, London

NHS Management Executive 1993 Day surgery report by the Day Surgery Task Force. HMSO, London, p. 9

Nelson S 1995 Preadmission clinics for thoracic surgery. Nursing Times 91(15): 29–31

Royal College of Surgeons of England 1992 Commission on the Provision of Surgical Services: guidelines for day case surgery. p. 8

Preparation for procedures

Eileen Lock

2

■ CONTENTS

OVERVIEW

To achieve the best out of day surgery, from the perspective of both patient and provider, patients must be appropriately selected and carefully prepared. This chapter will discuss aspects of preparation for day surgery that can have a positive influence on outcome.

Day surgery can demonstrate a high degree of patient satisfaction, as noted in the UK Audit Commission's research into day surgery, and patients' perceptions of service consistently show high levels of patient satisfaction.

Patients return to their own surroundings, which alleviates the stress of being in unfamiliar territory, thereby helping to accelerate recovery. The risk of developing a nosocomial (hospital acquired) infection is reduced by a shorter hospital stay. Financial savings made on funding inpatient beds can be concentrated into treating more patients, resulting in a more efficient service.

GENERAL FACTORS AFFECTING PREPARATION

Preparation of patients undergoing day surgery, after suitability of candidate has been clearly demonstrated, must take into account the following needs:

- physical
- intellectual
- emotional
- social.

Preparation for procedures needs to begin from the moment the patient consults his GP. The GP may advise the patient that he needs to have an operation or procedure carried out and refer him to a hospital consultant for treatment. The stress of the impending operation will begin to grow in the patient's mind. A multitude of questions may arise as a result: e.g.

- Is it serious?
- What are the complications?
- What if I don't come round from the anaesthetic?
- Who will look after the children/the home?
- Who will care for me?
- Can I take/afford time off from work?
- How will I manage?

Patients may experience physiological changes as a response to stress – and so, the pattern is set. If such patients are managed effectively and sensitively, their stresses and anxieties can be minimized by systematic preparation. This preparation must be synchronized by the multidisciplinary team. Information given to patients should be consistent from all of the staff encountered, to give credence to its content.

The point at which the day surgery nurse first comes into contact with the patient will vary from hospital to hospital. As far as day surgery is concerned, this, unfortunately, may not be until the day of surgery. Many hospitals have developed preadmission clinics or nurse assessment clinics, to meet patient needs. In hospitals with this facility, again the time at which the patient attends is variable. Many hospitals operate on a system whereby they invite patients to attend for preadmission clinics 2–4 weeks prior to surgery. This would appear to be an optimal time for both the patient and the personnel involved in her management, for the following reasons.

1. Any investigation which needs to be undertaken, such as Hb or ECG, would still be valid within a time span of 2–4 weeks.
2. Should the patient be seen too far in advance of the admission date, the surgery proposed may not be imminent enough to have enabled the patient to form an opinion or express fears/concerns. Thus, if the patient is seen too far in advance, as the date for day surgery approaches, her anxieties increase and time will not afford the opportunity to discuss those fears. This situation, in turn, does not provide the hospital staff the chance to allay these fears. The patient may subconsciously feel let down if the facility or forum to voice concerns has not been available. It is difficult to gain the confidence of the patient under these circumstances.

To fully prepare a patient for the prospect of undergoing surgery the nurse needs to be able to empathize with the patient's situation. Sometimes, for nursing professionals, it can become all too easy to forget how 'alien' the environment can seem to patients – in particular the language used. For example, 'Do you have any prosthesis?' may be met with an incredulous expression. Paradoxically, there is almost a need for the nurse to 'forget' everything she knows, to be able to give a helpful summary of what to expect in day surgery and what the procedure entails, and thus to gain the patient's confidence.

To give information to patients effectively, one needs to have a rudimentary understanding of how learning is achieved. In the case of the nurse–patient relationship, it must be borne in mind that individuals learn in different ways and gravitate to a particular style of learning based on past experience, heredity and environmental demands (Kolb 1988).

For health education/information to be effective, patients need to be given an active role. Emphasis needs to be placed on the patient's right to be fully informed. The Patient's Charter (DOH 1995) establishes the right of every citizen to be given a clear explanation of any treatment proposed under the National Health Service, including any risks and alternatives, before deciding whether they agree to treatment (see Chapter 8).

Educating patients, reported Wilson-Barnett (1983), can be defined as a process of increasing patients' understanding about their health, treatment and rehabilitation by giving information in a planned and structured way. The subject matter must be relevant to the needs of the individual patient. Verbal information should always be supplemented with good, clear, written information. Patients need a reference to which they can return to clarify instructions. It has been demonstrated by Gregor (1981) that patients who had received written information achieved higher knowledge scores in both short- and long-term evaluation.

> Verbal information to patients should always be supplemented with good, clear, written information.

Teaching should be a two-way communication between teacher and patient (Wilson-Barnett 1985). The teacher, i.e. the day surgery nurse, first needs to establish what the actual needs of the patient are. Involvement of the patient, by the nurse, with clear explanations and rationale for practice will increase the likelihood of successful learning and encourage the patient to seek further information. A well-informed patient, it can be concluded, is a less anxious patient. It has been demonstrated that the provision of preoperative information lowers anxiety levels, reduces stress and decreases pain and promotes a better and quicker recovery. Teaching specific activities that patients can undertake gives them a positive role to play in their own recovery, thereby increasing patient satisfaction (Boore 1978).

The reasons for non-compliance with given instructions are many and varied; pain, anxiety, fear, lack of knowledge and skills on the part of the teacher may all play a part. Research in this area by Dracup et al (1984) has shown that improved compliance can be achieved by simplifying instructions. The process of preparation prior to surgery should follow a well-recognized pattern:

- Assess
- Plan
- Implement
- Evaluate.

Assessment. Assessment of the patient's general health should be undertaken. This is best performed using a standardized questionnaire to ensure consistency and provide a framework on which to build. In addition to mutual discussion of the patient's needs, the medical notes should be used, in conjunction with the information given by the patient, to ensure a complete history is taken which will assist in planning care. A skilled assessor will be able to determine the patient's understanding and level of insight into their proposed treatment. The patient's perception of what is going to happen is very important at this stage, as it serves as a guide to how much, or how little, information needs to be further imparted by the nurse. Social support and home circumstances will also need to be established.

Planning. A plan of care should be made by the nurse with the co-operation of the patient, because patients tend to act in the light of what they themselves perceive as important. Conflict may arise when the nurse and the patient have differing perceptions of what is required or important.

Implementation. This involves putting the agreed care plan into action; these should have all relevant interventions documented.

Evaluation. Outcomes need to be evaluated to ascertain that what was planned for the patient was required, beneficial or, indeed, correct. Patient feedback is the most reliable form of determining patient satisfaction and success of planned care.

> A plan of care should be made by the nurse with the cooperation of the patient.

Allaying patients' anxieties

Few patients anticipate surgery without some degree of anxiety. Anxieties will vary from patient to patient but, in general, most arise from fear of pain, fear of anaesthetics, worries about family, dependants and coping with the mechanisms needed to facilitate hospital admission. For some patients the admission for day surgery will be their first time spent in hospital. Indeed, the criteria by which patients are selected for day surgery almost guarantee that we are dealing with otherwise fit and functional individuals.

Many patients will have young families. The coordination needed to ensure that the family is cared for alongside the ordeal of a hospital admission can add further stress to an already daunting situation.

For some patients it will always be seen as frightening – a journey into the unknown – and physiological changes may take place, such as a rise in heart rate, as a response to the stressful situation. This is more marked if the stress is prolonged. The preadmission clinic visit by the patient should be carefully planned to make it conducive to exchanging information. The interaction between nurse and patient should be conducted in a private room without fear of interruption. Patients often wish to discuss intimate or embarrassing issues and feel inhibited in doing so if they think they may be overheard. Adequate time must be set aside for this interview, and patients should be made to feel as relaxed as possible about using this time. The nurse should aim to create the ethos of being willing to assist with problems experienced by the patient as well as being able to empathize. During the preadmission visit, a first impression will have been formed by the patient. It is imperative that the confidence of the patient is gained and that the first impression is a favourable one.

Patients often have fears that are based on misinformation and misconception. The patient should be given a clear indication of what her proposed surgery will entail. A realistic guide should be given as to:

> For a preadmission visit, the interaction between nurse and patient should take place in a private room where the patient will feel able to discuss intimate issues.

- wound size and site;
- type of suturing material likely to be used;
- bandages, dressings, slings, crutches;

- recovery time needed (it is neither wise nor helpful to understate this, as patients need to make plans on the basis of the information given to them);
- pain/discomfort and methods of alleviation.

The nurse should also try to increase the patient's awareness as to degree of immobility that might be expected. Provided patients have this information in advance, they can generally cope very well. A maxim of openness and honesty is desirable.

PREADMISSION VISITS

Investigations which need to be taken prior to surgery will be organized at the preadmission clinic. This will help ensure that the results are analysed and dealt with accordingly. It should also dispense with the unsafe practice of switching the order of the operating list whilst awaiting the result of a hastily taken Hb, for example. Pre-admission preparation can enhance the quality of service not only to the patient but also to the multidisciplinary team of staff.

Another benefit that can be gained by patients from preadmission visits is that they can visualize exactly where they will be accommodated and can observe and familiarize themselves with the surroundings and the staff. They are also useful for explaining to relatives and carers where to come for collection. Patients do worry incessantly about the ability of their relatives to find the day surgery ward – even if it is well signposted!

Patients therefore benefit from being given a comprehensive guide to the day surgery ward. This should sequence events from admission to discharge. In briefing the patient, attention needs to be paid to the fine details, such as opening hours, telephone numbers and parking arrangements. The patient should be advised on what to bring on the day of admission. Many admission booklets now given to day surgery patients are exemplary in their design and content – probably as a response to demand. *Often, quality of care can still be enhanced by listening to what patients say they need.*

Regular, organized, critical review of nursing activity is desired to maintain efficiency. Patient satisfaction surveys need to be carried out frequently and on large sample numbers to sustain the highest standards. Staff must never allow themselves to become complacent once a satisfactory standard has been achieved. The whole process of care needs constant review to ensure change is instigated in response to demand.

Patients who smoke should be advised to stop, or at least reduce the number of cigarettes smoked in the weeks prior to surgery. Smoking is irritant to the respiratory tract and encourages secretions which may predispose the patient to respiratory complications during or after anaesthesia. If the nurse can provide a rationale, this will then enable the patient to understand the motives behind the request and help him to feel more responsible, which, in turn, should increase compliance.

> Patients benefit from being given a comprehensive guide to the day surgery ward and from being told all that will happen on their day of admission. Patients should be given details such as opening hours, telephone numbers and parking arrangements, and should be told what to bring with them. Nurses should listen to what patients say they need.

Paediatric patients

For this group the nurse has the role of reassuring both the child and the parent/guardian. As far as reasonable, the parent should be accommodated in the planning of care for the child's admission to hospital.

Policies as to whether the parent may accompany the child into the anaesthetic room will be in place locally, with the great majority of anaesthetists embracing this practice. The parent should be informed of any restrictions before the day of surgery – however, most day surgery wards are very much in favour of 'carer' involvement. It may be useful to remind parents that the child may bring a favourite toy, book or 'comforter' to the hospital.

Finally, something that may be overlooked is the need to advise the parent that they might need another person to accompany them home, especially if the parent is the driver. The child will most likely need to be comforted or held, which would make driving an impossibility (see Chapter 6).

> Most anaesthetists allow a parent to accompany a child into the anaesthetic room. The child may bring a favourite toy, book or 'comforter' to the hospital. The parent may need another person to accompany them home.

Patients who are to have a general anaesthetic on the day of surgery

The patient will have received a letter inviting them to attend for day surgery. The date, time and place of admission will be included along with other information. A map should be included to assist relatives/carers in finding the day surgery ward. As a measure of good practice, most day care units now send out a booklet outlining information relating to opening hours of the ward, telephone numbers, etc. The booklet may also be used to reinforce information given by the outpatient or preadmission clinics. It should also list items that the patient is required to bring along, such as:

- dressing gown
- slippers
- any tablets, inhalers or medication currently being used
- books or magazines
- small change, for the telephone
- toys, games or books, for children.

Patients should be reminded to leave their valuables and jewellery at home. They should also be reminded to avoid wearing make-up or nail varnish on the day of admission. Fasting times should be specified, as should the necessity to have an able and responsible person to escort the patient home and provide care in the first 24 hours following surgery.

Fasting

Fasting prior to surgery will need to be discussed with the patient before her date for admission. When undergoing surgery entailing general anaesthetic, the patient will need to have an empty stomach to prevent gastric contents being aspirated in the perioperative stage. Much has been written and researched on optimal fasting times, and there appears to be a great variance between hospitals. A generally accepted rule (Ogg & Hitchcock 1993) is that food should not have been consumed within 6 hours preoperatively and that clear oral fluids can be taken up to 3 hours before

> Patients should be told to consume no food for 4–6 h, and no liquid for 2–3 h, preoperatively. They should neither chew gum nor suck sweets during the fasting period.

elective surgery. However, it is becoming more common practice for food to be withheld for 4 hours and fluids for 2.

Patients sometimes mistakenly believe they can chew gum or suck sweets in the fasting period as they are not 'swallowing' anything. On the contrary, this can be a potentially dangerous action as chewing stimulates the secretion of gastric juices; gastric acidity therefore increases making vomiting more likely; gastric acidity may clear with a drink of water.

PREPARATION ON THE DAY OF SURGERY

Arrival at hospital

On the day of surgery the patient reports to the day surgery ward. In most cases the initial greeting will be from the clerical staff. It is essential that the patient is greeted in a calm and efficient manner, as often a patient's perception of events to come will be influenced by this first encounter. The patient should be introduced to the ward and the nurse or nursing members assigned to care for the patient. The nurse will welcome the patient, make an introduction and then orientate the patient to the ward. The patient will usually be interested to discover where the toilets, telephones and call-bell systems are located. The nurse will need to 'admit' the patient to the ward, which entails asking a number of questions, including those of a personal nature. The nurse should first explain to the patient that a number of questions need to be asked. This interview should be conducted in a quiet and private place to safeguard the privacy and dignity of the patient. Essential details such as name, address, date of birth, next of kin, hospital number and name of GP should be checked for accuracy. The patient will be given an identification bracelet bearing these details, to wear.

> It is essential that the patient is greeted in a calm and efficient manner.

The nurse then ascertains what level of understanding the patient has of the proposed surgery or procedure. The nurse should give the patient plenty of opportunity to ask questions and should attempt to clarify any uncertainties the patient may have.

The next step is to ensure that the patient has a suitable person to escort him home and provide the first 24 hours of care following surgery. The criteria for day surgery discharge states that the transport to home should be in a car. A postoperative patient is not a suitable candidate for public transport – the waiting time may precipitate dizziness or nausea, and fellow passengers are unlikely to notice or make allowance for infirmity. The name and contact number of the patient's escort to home should be documented in the nursing notes.

> The nurse should ensure that the patient has a suitable escort home; transport should be in a car.

The patient and her carer should be given some indication of a time when discharge home would be feasible. If this cannot be given, the carer should be encouraged to telephone the ward at a given time when this information would be available. Relatives of patients undergoing surgery experience as much stress as the patient, particularly during the intra-operative period (Lesky 1993). The nurse must include the needs of the relatives (as they will undoubtedly have an impact on the recovery of the patient) in the planning of care.

Information to and from patients

When did the patient last eat or drink?

Fasting. The patient will be asked when they last ate or drank. The time is recorded in the nursing notes. Patients often question the necessity of fasting. The admitting nurse should have a good understanding of the rationale behind preoperative fasting and offer the patient a sound explanation.

A study by Thomas (1983) found that 76% of patients were unaware of the reasons for fasting, and 62% unsure of the duration of fasting.

Is the patient taking medication?

Medication. The patient will be asked on the day of surgery if they are currently taking any medication. The drugs will be listed in the nursing notes. It should be verified that essential medication, such as antihypertensive drugs, has been taken. In the case of medically controlled diabetic patients, they will be advised to omit their medication during the period of fasting and recommence once normal eating and drinking is resumed. Diabetic patients will have a blood glucose analysis performed preoperatively and will be regularly monitored.

The patient must remove jewellery.

Jewellery. The nurse will ensure that the patient has removed all jewellery. The risks of diathermy can be negated by applying occluding tape to metallic objects. Another reason is that necklaces or watches may hinder a patient who suddenly needs to be turned onto their side in the recovery period.

The patient must remove make-up and nail varnish.

Make-up and nail varnish. Make-up and nail varnish need to be removed prior to surgery. The patient will be visually observed for signs of cyanosis (in addition to mechanical monitoring) in the postoperative period; thus it is essential that skin, lips and nails are not daubed by artificial colour. The extremities are the first to show signs of oxygen deprivation and therefore a crucial 'tool' for monitoring in the recovery phase.

Does the patient have any prostheses?

Prostheses. Patients are asked if they have any prostheses, e.g. pacemaker or joint replacements. A pacemaker would, in theory, rule out the patient as a suitable candidate for day surgery – however, it is prudent to double check. Joint replacements will be documented in the nursing notes. Patients who have had joint replacements often need to be placed in modified positions for surgery to avoid putting undue stress on the replaced joint.

The patient must remove contact lenses.

Contact lenses. Patients who wear contact lenses are advised that they will be required to remove them prior to going into the operating theatre. There is no need to remove them on arrival at the ward, as patients need to be able to read the consent form. Also, if they are waiting, they may appreciate being able to read a book or magazine.

Does the patient have any dentures, bridges, crowns or loose teeth?

Teeth. Patients are asked if they have any dentures, bridges, crowns or loose teeth; this information is then documented. In the case of dentures, they will need to be removed; this can be left until the patient is going into the operating theatre. Patients who wear dentures are generally very 'sensitive' about this requirement, and the dignity of the patient should be upheld.

Has the patient given consent?

Consent. The nurse will note if the patient has given informed consent to the operation or procedure that is to be carried out.

Sensitivities/allergies. Patients are asked if they have any allergies or sensitivities to drugs, plasters or any other substance. These should be highlighted in the patients' records.

Vital signs. Observations of blood pressure, pulse, temperature, respiration and weight should be taken and recorded. Weight is of particular importance in children as drug calculations are often determined on bodyweight.

The nurse admitting the patient should then proceed to give an account of the events of the day, explaining the requirement to change into an operating gown before going into surgery, and where the patient can store belongings. The patient will also be made aware that both the surgeon and anaesthetist may wish to consult and, inevitably, some questions may be duplicated. Although patients may find this exasperating, an explanation that the questioning is a safety measure, and reassurance that everyone is communicating and working as a team, should suffice.

It must be borne in mind, however, that patients will be anxious and therefore less able to retain information. Nyamthi & Kashiwabara (1988) evaluated the effects of preoperative anxiety on day surgery patients' ability to retain information and think constructively. They found 25% of patients to have high anxiety scores, with direct correlation of decreased ability to retain information as anxiety increased. Information given verbally, therefore, needs to be supplemented with written information.

Procedure-specific information sheets should be given out to patients, detailing dressings to be used, sutures and expected outcome. A contact telephone number should be given to patients as they may need further information after their discharge home. This helps to reassure patients that, once their surgery has been completed and they are safely back home, they are still welcome to contact us for advice and guidance.

Nurses need the skill to be able to adjust the 'pitch' of the preoperative briefing to suit the patient's level of understanding. Although all patients need accurate information to allay anxiety and to enable them to participate in their care, some patients will comprehend 'full' explanations better than others. Some patients are better able to vocalize exactly what they wish to know, others may struggle and, perhaps, keep silent. The nurse should study the body language and facial expressions of the patient to gauge if overload of information has occurred. It is important to prepare patients for their initial recovery period by explaining that blood pressure and pulse will be monitored frequently and that an oxygen mask may be placed on their face to deliver oxygen. It is paramount to emphasize that this is all normal and not an indication of problems.

Is the patient sensitive or allergic to drugs, plasters, etc.?

Vital signs should be recorded.

A procedure-specific information sheet should be given to the patient, detailing dressings, sutures and expected outcome, and providing a contact telephone number.

Pain

One of the most frequently worried-about aspects of surgery from the patients' perspective is pain. Pain can be defined as a distressing sensation caused by injury or disease. Pain, however, is a complex issue involving more than emotional, sensory and cognitive stimuli. The initial point at which a stimulus elicits the awareness of pain, is known as the 'pain threshold'.

Assessment of the experience of pain is essential for evaluating pain control strategies which need to be taken. Pain is extremely difficult to measure, as only the person experiencing it knows its nature and intensity. It may be helpful to patients if a visual display chart is used to measure pain. Observation of the patient should include vital signs, verbal responses (or lack of them), facial expressions, and other observations, e.g. restlessness, drawing up of knees, and thrashing movements.

> Giving patients preoperative information about postoperative pain lessens their anxiety.

A study by Rice & Johnson (1984) demonstrated that patients who have been given information about the type of sensations that they can expect to experience during a procedure have less fear and anxiety during the procedure. Information about anticipated pain sensations and what will be done to prevent or alleviate the pain, alters perception of pain although the pain stimuli remain unchanged. It has been indicated that the early provision of analgesia reduced postoperative problems.

Early administration of analgesia and regular evaluation of efficacy are needed to manage postoperative pain. Patients must be made aware before surgery that pain control is easier to achieve if commenced early rather than waiting until pain becomes unbearable. This information will, it is hoped, assist patients in reporting pain promptly.

Postoperative pain, particularly pelvic pain, is thought to trigger postoperative nausea and vomiting.

Postoperative nausea and vomiting

> One third of patients experience some degree of postoperative nausea and vomiting.

At least a third of all patients undergoing surgery experience some degree of postoperative nausea and vomiting. Typically this lasts up to 24 hours after surgery but may last as much as 48 hours in severe cases. Patients may experience between one and five episodes of vomiting. The harmful effects of postoperative nausea and vomiting can impact in several ways:

- discomfort and distress to patient
- embarrassment of patients at their perceived 'lack of control'
- tiredness caused by the physical energy expended in vomiting
- dehydration due to loss of fluids
- interference to electrolyte balance
- admission overnight for persistent nausea and vomiting.

The experience of postoperative nausea and vomiting can alter patients' attitudes to otherwise successful surgery. In a survey of day case patients by Madej & Simpson (1986), in the group of patients who were dissatisfied with the outcome of their operation, 71% cited postoperative nausea and vomiting as the reason.

Postoperative nausea and vomiting is up to three times more likely in a patient who has suffered previously; and so it must be noted at assessment.

Fasting for at least 6 hours prior to surgery (solid food) will help to avoid vomiting and regurgitation during or after anaesthesia. Stomach emptying, however, may be delayed as a result of anxiety, pain or hypotension, among other factors.

Movement of the patient postoperatively should be kept to a minimum. Transportation of the patient on a hospital trolley or bed should be managed as quietly and smoothly as possible.

Shaving

Preoperative shaving remains a controversial topic. Some surgeons have dispensed with the need for shaving, whereas others refuse to operate if shaving has not been carried out. This is a matter of local policy and negotiation. If shaving is required, it is best done as near to the surgery time as possible in order to reduce the possibility of bacterial growth.

Local anaesthesia

Local anaesthesia involves the surgical site's being infiltrated with an agent, such as lignocaine, to make the area numb. Patients undergoing operation under local anaesthesia will be equally as anxious as those undergoing general anaesthesia, and will require the same degree of psychological support and preparation.

Explanation of the procedure should be detailed, as the patient will be awake in the operating room. The nurse caring for the patient should endeavour to make the patient feel as secure as possible in relation to the pending surgery. A description of the operating room and references to who would be available to assist all play a part in reassuring the patient. It is important to convey to the patient that he will not be left alone and that throughout the procedure there will be a named person responsible.

THE NURSE'S ROLE IN HEALTH EDUCATION AND PROMOTION IN THE DAY SURGERY SETTING

Many people may assume that patients undergoing day surgery are not in hospital long enough for the opportunity of health education to arise. This is a serious misconception. The day surgery nurse plays a major role in this aspect of nursing. A discussion regarding health status and lifestyle progresses naturally as the nurse is assessing or preparing patients for surgery. It is the ideal opportunity for further exploration of individual needs regarding health education or information. It is part of the role of every nurse to aid and assist individuals in taking responsibility for their health. As far back as 1859, Florence Nightingale stated that 'nursing has been limited to signify little more than the administration of medicines and the application of poultices. It ought to signify the proper use of fresh air, light, warmth, cleanliness, quiet and the proper selection and administration of diet'. This statement advocating a more proactive role by the nurse in giving advice about healthy living shows that health education is not a newly discovered concept in the nursing world.

The day surgery nurse can play a major role in health education.

The day surgery nurse needs to have the ability to assess the suitability of patients for day surgery. To do this effectively, the nurse needs to be aware of what might be considered a health risk. A nurse working in the day surgery environment will be only too aware of the negative aspects of obesity, hypertension, smoking, alcohol abuse and stress – to name but a few. In order to discuss such issues with the patient, the nurse must have some understanding of methods of improving or optimizing health.

The nurse in the day surgery will often be approached by the patient for information. Patients will expect the nurse to be able to provide this. A resourceful nurse should be aware of supplementary providers of health education. The nurse is not expected to have all the answers, but there is no reason why the patient cannot be guided to refer to other sources for information. For example, a patient coming into hospital for the removal of a breast lump might seek further advice on aftercare. The nurse would be able to provide the patient with leaflets on breast self-examination and breast awareness as well as discussing the general care surrounding this particular operation. In addition the nurse could also provide the contact telephone number of the breast care clinical specialist. This person would be equipped to give more in-depth information and, should the lump prove malignant, counselling and future support. The day surgery nurse does not need to be a walking encyclopedia on health education and promotion, but should know what other help is available and how to make contact. For reference purposes a regularly updated directory can be maintained on the day surgery ward.

The World Health Organization (WHO) stated in 1978 that people have the right to be involved in both the planning and the implementation of their healthcare, including health education. Health promotion and health education are not the same. Health education provides patients with information to make an informed choice. Health promotion encompasses all aspects of a total health package: screening, immunization, school health checks. Health education, therefore, is only a part of the much broader issue of health promotion. The nurse in the day surgery setting promotes the health of the patient by giving health education which is a valuable input to the wider spectrum of healthcare. The quality of the information given must be research-based, user friendly and accurate.

Health education leaflets are readily available in most day surgery wards. Attractive displays of leaflets on a variety of health topics could prove of interest to patients. Information leaflet displays need to be maintained regularly to ensure interest is sustained by the patients. People do not need to be coerced into health education, but eye-catching displays or posters will often capture added interest. It could be argued that the general public appear to have developed an insatiable appetite for anything relating to health issues. It seems that the media too are on this particular bandwagon. But if it enhances the public awareness of health issues, so much the better.

Should a patient seek help on an issue relating to health, it may be considered as the first step towards increasing knowledge and understanding and taking control and should be encouraged with a well-structured response; therefore:

- Ascertain exactly what is being asked.
- Establish what is already known.
- Negotiate a desired outcome.
- Facilitate the patient's achievement of the desired outcome.

REFERENCES

Boore J 1978 Prescription for recovery. Royal College of Nursing, London
DOH 1995 The Patient's charter and you. Department of Health, London
Dracup et al 1984 Group counselling in cardiac rehabilitation: effect on patient compliance. Patient Education and Counselling 6(4): 169–177
Gregor F M 1981 Teaching the patient with ischaemic heart disease – a systematic approach to instruction design. Patient Counselling and Health Education 3(2): 57–62
Kolb 1988 Patient education: a literature review. Journal of American Nursing 13: 203–213
Lesky J S 1993 Anxiety of elective surgical patients' family members – relationship between anxiety levels and family characteristics. AORN Journal 57(5): 1091–1101
Madej T H, Simpson K H 1986 Comparison of the use of domperidone, droperidol and metoclopromide in the prevention of nausea and vomiting following major abdominal and gynaecological surgery. British Journal of Anaesthetists 58: 884–887
Nyamthi A, Kashiwabara A 1988 Pre-operative anxiety. AORN Journal 47(1): 164–169
Ogg T W, Hitchcock M 1993 What is the optimum NPO time prior to day surgery. Journal of One-day Surgery (Summer): 4–5
Palazzo M G, Strunnin L 1984 Anesthesia and emesis II – prevention and management. Canadian Anesthetic Society Journal 31: 407–415
Rice V H, Johnson J E 1984 Pre-admission self instruction booklets: post-admission exercise programme and teaching time. Nursing Research 33(3): 147–151
Thomas E A 1983 Pre-operative fasting: a question of routine? Nursing Times 49: 46–47
Wilson-Barnett J 1983 Patient teaching. Churchill Livingstone, Edinburgh
Wilson-Barnett J 1985 Principles of patient teaching. Nursing Times 81(8): 28–29

Operating room practice

3

Eve Unerman

Nursing practice in the operating room (OR) of a day surgery unit (DSU) follows very much the same principles as those for a large operating department. Health and safety, infection control, handling and lifting, and care planning are essential to the production of quality nursing care in both areas. Probably the main difference between the two areas is the patient. In day care surgery the patient is in reasonable health and quite often is awake for the whole of his procedure. A bonus regarding care planning in a DSU is the juxtaposition of the pre- and postoperative care areas to the operating room in those units that are self-contained. This benefits both patients and staff.

To facilitate the safe passage of a patient through the OR it is necessary to provide a safe environment. To achieve this the following aspects require consideration:

- health and safety
- handling and lifting
- infection control
- staff education

HEALTH AND SAFETY

Health and safety in the work place is defined in the UK by the Health and Safety at Work Act, 1974. This act provides legislative power to promote the safety, health and welfare of a working environment and those that are required to work in this environment. It is described as a parent act in that further legislation may be added to it at later dates. These additions take the form of Regulations, Codes of Practice, and European Directives, and are added to the parent act as and when new industry or practice arises. To ensure health and safety at work an employer is required to provide protocols or guidelines for safe practice. The employee is required to adhere to and implement these guidelines, following any necessary education and training (Chard, 1993).

Guidelines issued by NATN (National Association of Theatre Nurses) on the promotion of safe practice in the OR will contain elements of the Health and Safety at Work Act, 1974 as will those issued by NHS Trusts and Health Authorities. Fairchild (1993) bases a great deal of her discussion of the OR environment on standards and recommended practices set by AORN (Association of Operating Room Nurses) as well as state directives. To achieve safety in the OR, fundamental policies are deployed, but these will also be combined with research, knowledge and experience to achieve care of a high standard.

The recommended size of an OR is about $20 \times 20 \times 10$ ft ($6.5 \times 6.5 \times 3$ m) to provide a minimum floorspace of 360 ft^2 (about 40 m^2) (Fairchild 1993). Papa Petros (1994) gives a dimension for major rooms in a DSU as 24×24 ft (576 ft^2 or about 60 m^2). Whatever the minimum recommended size, it is necessary to take into consideration the amount of furniture and equipment that may be required both now and in the future. Fairchild (1993) lists the following equipment as being essential for patient and staff safety:

- a communications system
- oxygen and vacuum outlets
- mechanical ventilation assistance equipment
- respiratory and cardiac monitoring equipment
- X-ray illumination boxes
- air filters
- adequate lighting
- emergency lighting system
- cardiac defibrillator (share with unit).

Add to this list the actual furniture required, e.g. the operating table, trolleys, suction equipment, positioning aids, a diathermy machine, stools, plus any further specialist equipment, and the available space is soon filled. All equipment and furniture is required to be checked on a regular basis to ensure fitness for function, i.e. that a particular piece of furniture is safe to use as prescribed by the Health and Safety at Work Act, 1974 (Chard 1993).

HANDLING AND LIFTING

Approximately 70% of people will suffer from low back pain at some time during their lives. Those in manual occupations are more likely to suffer from back pain than those whose work is less demanding, although there are other factors to consider such as the amount of time spent sitting, standing, twisting or bending.

Onset of pain may be acute or insidious with a buildup of damage over a period of time. Even with an acute attack it is quite often difficult to identify the actual factor that caused the damage, because of this buildup. On the whole, people with a back injury tend to experience pain in one of two ways:

1. intermittent episodes of pain with intervals symptom free
2. continual pain, never quite symptom free.

Problems arise when damage done exceeds rate of recovery (Pheasant 1991).

The RCN Code of Practice for the Handling of Patients, updated in 1993, was produced to reduce the incidence of back and other injuries to nurses. The Code is relevant for the handling of equipment and loads as well as patients. It also takes into account the recommendations of an EC directive which have been incorporated into the Manual Handling Operations Regulations (1992). The RCN Code is divided into three sections:

1. the management of people – the employers' responsibilities
2. the management of self – the employee's responsibilities
3. the management of patients and clients – assessment and the planning of care.

From this legislation two concepts have been identified (RCN 1993):

- The employer has the statutory duty to assess every task requiring lifting or manual handling.
- There is a need to apply ergonomic principles to the planning and organization of patient handling.

A study by Addington (1994) discusses a programme devised to reduce the incidence of back injuries in OR nurses (including those from the DSU). This programme came about as a result of an initiative of the occupational health department at her hospital, who devised and implemented a 'Ready, Steady, Lift' programme to highlight prevention of injury. Each clinical area was required to send a key person to intensive workshops to become the 'back trainer' for their area. When the OR trainers (one of whom was Addington) tried to implement what they had learned into their area, they found that OR staff members identified activities other than patient handling that caused back pain.

These activities included:

- pushing/pulling
- bending/twisting
- carrying
- over-reaching
- handling equipment
- standing for prolonged periods
- holding retractors
- walking on hard floors.

The trainers were then able to develop the following recommendations:

- *correct posture* – practice shifting weight if standing for long periods; pivot rather than twist the body at the waist to reach materials; wear shock-absorbing footwear in the absence of fatigue-absorbing floor covering;
- *education* – video and self-assessment manual followed by discussion to reinforce positive practice; use of a pre- and post-test to increase effectiveness; validation of programme by observation of employee at work to check on correct performance;

Practice shifting weight if standing for long periods. Pivot rather than twist the body at the waist to reach materials.

- *fitness* – as muscle weakness is implicated in injury (Braggins 1994), a fitness consultant was called in to advise, and the result was that the department acquired two exercise bikes for the use of the staff, which proved immensely popular!
- *enlist help of others* – OH department and physiotherapists asked to advise and support the programme and the staff.

Evaluation of the programme a year later indicated an increased awareness of back injury prevention generally. The staff were wearing recommended shoes, fewer days were taken off sick with back pain, fitness and health increased, as did the number of handling devices purchased by the department. Addington in her conclusion feels that the programme had been a success and will continue to be so as long as there is a daily commitment. She says 'We now realize that taking care of our backs is a 24 hour job'.

Gamble & Aires (1994) also found that maintaining health and safety in a theatre environment was a 24 hour activity requiring constant attention and updating. In response to the RCN Code (1993) they developed and used risk assessment techniques to promote healthy and safe working conditions. Some areas identified caused concern with regard to lifting and handling, with the potential for back injury. An example given was the handling of large oxygen cylinders on the patients' trolleys. Through assessment of the problem and the situation it was possible to fit smaller and lighter cylinders, so reducing the risk of injury. Gamble & Aires identified other areas of risk which resulted in changes to practice, reducing the potential for injury and at the same time improving patient care.

Within the OR the employer has the responsibility to ensure provision of correct handling aids and equipment that is suitable for its purpose – for example, the operating table. It is now possible to purchase patient trolleys that also double as the operating tale. This means that a patient remains on the same piece of equipment throughout their stay in the DSU, thus removing the need for transfer of the patient from trolley to table and back again with the attendant risk to patient and staff. The new patient trolleys are much easier to use being adjustable in height and easily manoeuvred. Wherever the patient is, the nurse caring for her is able to adjust the trolley to suit herself and the patient, so cutting out potentially harmful stooping and twisting. This is relevant for the nurse in anaesthetics and recovery as well as in the OR. Within the DSU the moving of patients prior to surgery is almost eliminated, as many patients walk into the OR and position themselves on the operating table before being anaesthetized.

Staff have an obligation to keep themselves updated regarding lifting and handling and to be knowledgeable about the use of equipment. Noting the work of Addington (1994) and Gamble & Aires (1994), OR staff should also have regard for their own working environment and for their health and general body awareness. Fitness is thought to help in the prevention of back injury (Braggins 1994). Fitness will also increase body awareness. A fit person is far more likely to be aware of the position of his body and what he is able to do in the way of twisting and bending.

Stress is implicated in back pain. Acute stress leads to muscle tension which, if prolonged over a period of time, could facilitate damage to the muscles of the back. In chronic stress, muscle fatigue could occur through a decrease in muscle caused by the glucocorticosteroid hormones (Clarke & Montague 1993). Psychological stress contributes to muscle tension. The tension occurs in different sets, sometimes characteristically, of muscles (Pheasant 1991). It seems that repressed anger could produce neck pain, whereas low back pain may be associated with anxiety.

Tension on a set of muscles may then affect the posture of a person, who may exert tension on other sets of muscles in an effort to balance the body. Another factor of stress that may be implicated in back pain is the length of time worked before taking a break. It seems that the more stressed a person is, the longer they will work without a break and the shorter the break is when they eventually take it. This builds up to chronic fatigue with the potential for back injury.

INFECTION CONTROL

Infection control is vital in the OR to prevent the spread and growth of pathogenic bacteria and viruses. Control is necessary in the interests of preserving the health of patients, staff and the environment. The following need to be controlled:

- ventilation
- temperature and humidity
- cleaning and sterilization
- clothing
- hand washing
- behaviour.

Ventilation

To reduce the possiblity of airborne contamination in the OR, an efficient ventilatory system is recommended. The number of microorganisms in the air depends on the size of the room, the amount of activity, the number of persons and the rate at which the air is replaced (Caddow 1989).

Room or indoor air contains microorganisms commonly found in the human respiratory tract. Coughing, talking and sneezing all cause bacteria, in some quantity, to be released into the air. Each infectious droplet so released loses its moisture by evaporation, leaving mucus and organic debris to which the bacteria remain attached. Dust is also capable of harbouring bacteria, as are skin scales shed as people move. *Staphylococcus aureus*, for example, is resistant to drying and is able to survive for long periods on dust particles (Brock et al 1994).

The OR is an enclosed space, partly to keep bacteria and other micro-organisms out. An efficient ventilation system not only ensures comfortable working conditions but aids in the removal of airborne particles. Current recommendations require 20–25 air changes per hour, with 5 of these being with clean air (Fairchild 1993, Caddow 1989). This will also prevent the buildup of air pollutants (Pheasant 1991). In the OR these pollutants could come from hazardous solutions and anaesthetic gases.

The airflow through the OR is maintained by positive pressure. This forces old air out of the room but prevents potentially contaminated air from entering. This system relies on all doors to and from the OR being closed except when actually in use (AORN 1993a).

Temperature and humidity

Temperature is one of the most important environmental factors influencing the growth and survival of microorganisms. With an increase in temperature there is a corresponding increase in the growth rate of the microorganism until a limit is reached. At lower temperatures the growth rate is slowed (Brock et al 1994). Pathogenic bacteria will tend to favour a warm, humid environment for growth, mimicking the internal environment of the body. Within the OR, to keep bacterial growth to a minimum, both temperature and humidity need to be controlled. The recommended temperature range is 20–24°C, whilst humidity should be maintained between 50% and 55% (Fairchild 1993). Controlling temperature and humidity also contributes to a comfortable working environment, although it is necessary to raise the temperature of the OR prior to paediatric surgery. Children lose heat rapidly since they have a relatively high body surface area and low body mass with little insulating subcutaneous fat (Joy 1990).

> Recommended range of temperature in the OR is 20–24°C; it is necessary to raise the temperature above normal prior to paediatric surgery. Humidity should be 50–55%.

Cleaning and sterilization

At the beginning of the day, before the start of any list, a procedure called 'damp dusting' is usually carried out, since removing dust should correspondingly help keep bacterial levels down. Mackrodt (1994) questioned the damp dusting tradition, but results indicated that damp dusting is useful in this respect. However, it is not easy to ascertain clearly the efficiency of damp dusting as there are several factors to consider – for example, the number of staff carrying out the procedure, the clothing they are wearing and the fabric type – which may cause an increase in dust levels and the bacterial count. Newer ORs with more efficient ventilation systems are less in need of damp dusting, since a good ventilation system removes debris more effectively. A DSU has to be assessed on these factors, to ascertain the necessity of damp dusting.

During the implementation of a theatre list, all furniture and equipment that has been in contact with a patient is considered contaminated and must be cleaned before use for the next patient; this includes mopping the floor. At the end of a list, all furniture and equipment in the OR must be cleaned and the floor scrubbed (Fairchild 1993). Use of hot water and detergent is sufficient to remove debris and render the equipment socially clean. Disinfectants are only required if an infected case has been treated. (Note the distinction between disinfectants, which are 'chemicals that kill microorganisms and are used on inanimate objects', and antiseptics, which are 'chemical agents that kill or inhibit growth of microorganisms and that are sufficiently nontoxic to be applied to living tissue' (Brock et al 1994).)

Following an infected case, the equipment is cleaned as usual, then the recommended disinfectant (as per hospital policy) is applied and left to dry. Usually, following cleaning, surfaces are dried to prevent the growth

> Disinfectants kill microorganisms and are used on inanimate objects. Antiseptics kill or inhibit growth of microorganisms and are sufficiently non-toxic to be applied to living tissue.

of microorganisms (Caddow 1989). Floors are wet scrubbed as this is less likely to cause the release of bacteria into the air. All mops and brushes used in the cleaning of the floor must be changed and cleaned after use (Fairchild 1993). She also recommends a long-term cleaning programme to allow for the thorough cleaning of the whole theatre suite.

Sterilization

Sterilization is the 'complete killing of all microorganisms' (Brock et al 1994). In other words, a product or article is sterile or it isn't. All microorganisms, including spores, must be destroyed during the sterilization process for an article to be described as sterile. Following proper packing, sealing and sterilization, an article may remain sterile for a considerable length of time. Method of storage affects sterility rather than the length of storage time (Fairchild 1993). Packaging does need to be checked for damage on a regular basis, and in some units there are guidelines on when articles and equipment are no longer deemed sterile.

Method of sterilization (see Box 3.1) depends on the product or article to be sterilized. The majority of instruments used in a theatre may be sterilized in an autoclave following decontamination. An autoclave is a sterilizer designed to use steam under pressure, allowing the steam to reach temperatures high enough to destroy microorganisms. The higher the temperature reached, the shorter is the cycle required to achieve sterilization (Fairchild 1993). Autoclaving is the preferred method for a theatre sterilization unit.

Delicate items such as catheters and other single-use items can be sterilized using gamma radiation. This method of sterilization is very expensive and is normally associated with commercially prepared items rather than in-house ones, since the cost would be too great for an individual hospital or Trust.

Chemical sterilization with ethylene oxide gas is expensive and requires a long sterilization cycle – 2 to 5 hours – as well as a lengthy period of time

---

■ **BOX 3.1 Methods of sterilization (adapted from Caddow 1989, Warren 1983)**

1. wet heat sterilization (using an autoclave)
   121°C for 15 min
   134°C for 3 min

2. low-temperature steam and formaldehyde
   72–80°C for 1–2 h

3. chemical sterilization with ethylene oxide
   50°C for 1–16 h
   (requires aeration period of 24 h)

4. irradiation
   2.5 Mrad required to ensure sterility (expensive to run; uses gamma rays – ionizing radiation)

thereafter to allow for aeration of items. This method can be used for instruments and equipment that are unable to withstand the high temperature and pressure of the autoclave. It is probably seldom used now, because of expense, the time required and the health and safety problems associated with using ethylene oxide.

Hand scrubbing

The purpose of the surgical hand scrub (AORN 1994a) is to:

1. remove debris and transient microorganisms from the finger nails, hands and forearms
2. reduce the resident microbial count to a minimum
3. inhibit rapid rebound growth of microorganisms.

The following recommendations are put forward by AORN in the interests of enhancing the scrub technique.

> Remove watches, rings and bracelets before scrubbing hands. Keep finger nails short, clean and healthy. Cuticles, hands and forearms should be free of open lesions and breaks in the skin.

1. Remove watches, rings and bracelets, as they may harbour microorganisms. Occasionally an allergic reaction may occur as a result of the scrub agent collecting underneath the jewellery.
2. Finger nails should be kept short, clean and healthy. Long nails can tear gloves and cause trauma to the patient. Nail varnish has not been shown to increase the bacterial count but chipped varnish that has been worn for longer than 4 days may pose a risk.
3. Cuticles, hands and forearms should be free of open lesions and breaks in skin integrity.

Ross (1994), whilst reviewing the literature for a research study, found that as long as a scrub technique using 'soap' and water was used for the first scrub, then subsequent 'scrubs' could be replaced by an alcohol rub. From the study undertaken, the following recommendations emerged.

1. Use spray taps to reduce water costs. These should be foot or knee operated.
2. The traditional scrub after first wash should be replaced by 70% isopropyl alcohol rub.
3. Pre-sterilized brushes are cheaper than resterilized and are safer.

Scrub agents should:

1. reduce microorganisms on intact skin
2. be broad spectrum
3. be fast acting or have a residual effect
4. be non-irritant
5. contain an antimicrobial agent.

The most common examples are chlorhexidine and Betadine. Betadine (providone iodine) is fast acting with a prolonged action. Iodine is present in very small concentrations, thus reducing the incidence of sensitization (Seaton Health Care Group plc).

The length of the scrub procedure should be between 3 and 5 minutes. Fairchild (1993) would claim that 5 minutes is necessary.

Clothing

Theatre clothing plays an important role in the control of infection. All clothing used in a theatre setting should be designed and manufactured to limit, as much as possible, the airborne spread of bacteria and other microorganisms. At the same time, clothing needs to be comfortable and easily laundered. Cost also needs consideration. Tunics and trousers are generally now worn by theatre personnel. These are comfortable and allow for ease of movement, an important ergonomic consideration. Dresses may be worn, but Fairchild (1993) maintains that if dresses are the preferred choice then the legs must be covered to prevent the shedding of skin scales. As well as design, choice of fabric is important. Fabrics used for the manufacture of tunics, trousers and dresses must be lint free (to reduce dust levels and therefore bacterial levels) and flame resistant (Fairchild 1993). Cotton is not a suitable fabric as it sheds fibres and is of an open weave, absorbing fluids rapidly and thus offering little protection against accidental spillage of fluids (Caddow 1987).

Similarly surgical gowns and patient drapes should be made of fabrics that repel water, are comfortable, safe and easy to use and minimize the amount of shedding that may occur from the skin and indeed the fabrics (AORN 1994).

The use of masks and head covering by all theatre personnel for every case is now questioned. Gould (1994) discusses research regarding this issue. The use of a mask does not appear to make any difference to the rate of infection. Following research into the use of masks, Mitchell & Hunt (1991) suggest that the routine use of masks is unnecessary. Oral dispersal of microorganisms during quiet speech is low, with a corresponding low risk of wound infection. Contamination of the wound by non-masked members of the scrub team can occur; therefore it is recommended that masks are worn by a scrub team performing high-risk surgery. Wearing of masks by non-scrubbed personnel is unnecessary. Orr & Bailey (1992) consider that the wearing of masks is not essential for routine general surgery; similarly the use of head coverings. It is recommended that non-scrubbed personnel not directly involved with the operating site do not need to cover their hair except in high-risk situations (Humphreys et al 1991). The above recommendations only apply in theatre suites that have an efficient ventilation system.

Behaviour

Behaviour of OR personnel will have an effect on infection control. Movement around the theatre, respecting the 'clean' and 'dirty' areas, keeping doors closed and actually minimizing movement all help to maintain a low bacterial count. Correct use and disposal of clothing, gowns, masks, gloves and headgear again can affect the level of microorganisms in the OR. Importantly, a good aseptic technique is required by all personnel. Asepsis, as defined by Burton (1992), is the 'absence of infectious microorganisms on living tissue'. Aseptic technique therefore is the process whereby all infectious microbes are removed or excluded from living tissues.

This requires the correct use of disinfectants, antiseptics and sterilization (Burton 1992).

It is now recommended that universal precautions should be practised for all invasive procedures (AORN 1992, Burton 1992). This is to protect personnel and patients from exposure to blood-borne pathogens such as hepatitis B virus and HIV. This includes the use of eye protection, gowns and gloves, although what is used depends on the level of involvement in care. Also recommended is the use of a hands-free technique when sharps are passed between personnel. Contaminated sharps need to be disposed of appropriately, as does any other waste, to prevent cross-infection. Universal precautions not only reduce the possibility of potential infection but they remove the possibility of discrimination of both patients and personnel who could be classed as 'infectious'.

Infection control for the perioperative nurse is a central issue of patient care (Rothrock 1990). Knowledge of microbiology and infection control procedures is vital for, although maintenance and regard of procedures are necessary, are they suitable for every patient that passes through the day surgery unit? The fitter the patient the less likely is she to contract an infection. Ayliffe et al (1992) discuss the 'fitness' of the patient for operation. Those patients that are at greater risk of infection tend to have spent some time in hospital prior to surgery, are obese, cachetic or have uncontrolled diabetes. These are patients that do not normally appear in the day surgery unit. The healthy patient needs to be taken into account when assessing and planning infection control measures, but this should be balanced with the need for universal precautions and recent research findings such as the use of masks and head coverings in the OR. This is why the perioperative nurse requires knowledge, to be able to plan the care of an individual effectively in spite of an ever-increasing amount of research, new products and information.

> Infection control for the perioperative nurse is a central issue of patient care. Knowledge of microbiology and infection control procedures is vital.

PLANNING OF CARE

Holistic patient care in the OR depends on the nurse's making correct decisions about the care that is required by the patient, based on his knowledge of the patient and his expert knowledge. Schober (1993), in discussing models of decision making, including the nursing process, comments on the importance to nurses of considering how decisions about care are made and what factors can affect these decisions. These factors include the sharing of power between nurse and patient to allow for exchange of information and the development of a therapeutic relationship. This will allow the patient to become involved in her care, another factor that can affect decision making. The process of assessment not only influences decisions but is the key to effective care planning (Schober 1993), where planning is 'the establishment of specific goals and/or outcome criteria for the individual patient' (Fairchild 1993).

Ideally, in the DSU each patient would have his own nurse who would carry out his assessment, plan care in collaboration with him, be part of the team(s) that implement the care and evaluate the care and its outcomes.

This would result in good, holistic perioperative care delivered by a perioperative nurse using the nursing process (Kleinbeck 1990). According to Kleinbeck (1990), 'perioperative' describes the period of time that includes before, during and immediately following surgery. In day surgery, in addition to the perioperative period there is also assessment and discharge planning to consider.

The development of a partnership between patient and nurse, with the nurse assuming responsibility for the care of the patient throughout her stay in hospital, is embodied in the principles of Primary Nursing (Black 1992). Within the DSU the role of the Primary Nurse could be integrated with that of Clinical Nurse Specialist. A Clinical Nurse Specialist not only is an expert practitioner in her area of practice but will also have increased her knowledge and skills through education. The role encompasses expert practice, research, education and a consultative role (Manley 1993). The Clinical Nurse Specialist in a DSU would be a specialist in all aspects of care in the unit, and it is feasible that there would be several nurses so employed (depending on the size of the unit). Within the OR this would ensure that a specialist nurse would be available to ensure that high standards of care are maintained. It would also ensure that care for each patient would be planned and supervised by one nurse, even though at times others may be carrying out the care.

STAFF EDUCATION

To be able to make informed decisions on patient care and staff safety within the operating room requires a constant updating of knowledge and skills. This is necessary to keep abreast of environmental and social changes as well as the advances and developments in day surgery itself. Changes in any of these areas could lead to a change in clinical practice if not to the environment of the operating room itself.

Infection control is not as straightforward as it may appear. Micro-organisms are constantly mutating, developing resistance to drugs as well as the potential for new infectious illnesses. Work-related stress and the devastating effects that this may have on an individual are now frequently reported in the newspapers. These are but two examples of why constant updating is necessary. Regular attendance on study days, some of which are now mandatory, e.g. Manual Handling, and specialist courses provide a means of keeping up with changes and developing practice to cope with them. On a day-to-day basis, maintenance of standards allows for safe practice. As well as updating, good practices can be established through thorough induction programmes for new staff and by encouraging people to read departmental/unit policies plus any additions to such policies when and if they occur.

This will help to promote the health and safety of all those, both patients and staff, who come into contact with the operating room, by giving the OR staff the knowledge as well as the skills to perform effectively in their work.

REFERENCES

Addington C 1994 All the right moves. AORN Journal 59(2): 483–488
AORN 1992 Proposed recommended practices (universal precautions). AORN Journal 56(1): 115–119
AORN Recommended Practices Committee 1993a Recommended practices: traffic patterns in the surgical suite. AORN Journal 57(3): 730–734
AORN Recommended Practices Committee 1993b Proposed recommended practices: environmental responsibilities in the practice setting. AORN Journal 57(4): 970–977
AORN Recommended Practices Committee 1994a Proposed recommended practices for surgical hand scrubs. AORN Journal 60(2): 270
AORN Recommended Practices Committee 1994b Proposed recommended practices for surgical attire. AORN Journal 60(2): 282–292
Atwell C 1990 Control of substances hazardous to health. Surgical Nurse (July). 10–13
Ayliffe G A J, Lowbury E J L, Geddes A, Williams J D 1992 Control of hospital infection. Chapman and Hall Medical, London
Black F (ed.) 1992 Primary nursing, an introductory guide. King's Fund Centre
Braggins S 1994 The back. Mosby Year Book Europe,
Brock T D, Madigan M T, Martenko J M, Parker J 1994 Biology of microorganisms, 7th edn. Prentice-Hall International, New Jersey
Burton G R 1992 Microbiology for the health sciences, 4th edn. J B Lippincott, Philadelphin
Chard C 1993 Health and safety for nurses. Chapman and Hall, London
Clarke E, Montague S 1993 The nature of stress and its implications for nursing practice. In: Hinchliff S M, Norman S E, Schober J E (eds) Nursing practice and health care, 2nd edn. Edward Arnold, London, ch 9
Fairchild S 1993 Perioperative nursing: principles and practice. Jones & Bartlett, Boston
Gamble P, Aires P 1994 Caring for health and safety counts. British Journal of Theatre Nursing 4(9): 5–9
Gould D 1994 Infection control in high risk environments. Nursing Standard 8(30): 57–61
Health and Safety Executive 1992 The manual handling operation regulations. HMSO, London.
Humphreys H, Russell A J, Ricketts V E, Reeves D S 1991 The effect of surgical head-gear on air bacterial counts. Journal of Hospital Infection 19: 175–180
Joy C 1990 Pediatric surgery. In: Rothrock J C (ed.) Perioperative nursing care planning, Mosby, London, ch 21
Kleinbeck S 1990 Introduction to the nursing process. In: Rothrock J C (ed.) Perioperative nursing care planning, Mosby, London, ch 1
Mackrodt K 1994 Damp dusting in the operating theatre: implications for bacteria counts. British Journal of Theatre Nursing 4(9): p. 10–13
Manley K 1993 The clinical nurse specialist. Surgical Nurse 6(3): 21–25
Mitchell N J, Hunt S 1991 Surgical face masks in modern operating rooms – a costly and unnecessary ritual? Journal of Hospital Infection 18: pp 239–242
Papa Petros P E 1994 Planning, building and operating a free-standing privately-owned day theatre complex: a nine year experience. Ambulatory Surgery 2: 39–42
Pheasant S 1991 Ergonomics, work and health. Macmillan,
Ross C 1994 What cost ritual? British Journal of Theatre Nursing 4(4): 11–14
Rothrock J C 1990 Perioperative nursing care planning. Mosby, London
RCN 1993 Code of practice for the handling of patients. Royal college of nursing, London.
Schober J 1993 Approaches to nursing care. In: Hinchliff S M, Norman S E, Schober J E (eds) Nursing practice and health care, 2nd edn. Edward Arnold, London, ch 8
Warren M C 1983 Operating theatre nursing. Lippincott Nursing Series, Harper & Row, London

Procedures undertaken in day surgery

Bernadette Phelan   Sarah Grenside

Day surgery is fast becoming one of the most successful alternatives in contemporary health care delivery systems. As a result of recent changes within the UK National Health Service (e.g. the greater need for financial restraint, increased patient throughput and cost competitiveness), day surgery offers great potential by allowing a large throughput of patients at a lower financial cost than inpatient care, without affecting the quality of care (Audit Commission 1991).

For the perioperative nurse there are opportunities to condense and refine traditional nursing skills and to develop a mindset that is specifically turned to wellness, safety, teaching and continuity of care. Day surgery enables perioperative nurses to be creative in their approach to patient care. Perioperative nursing can be optimally applied with day surgery patients because the entire care episode takes place in a short time. Continuity of care is provided through the perioperative, intraoperative and the postoperative phase of the patient's stay.

Hutching (1995) states that technical advances in surgery and anaesthesiology now permit many surgical procedures, which formerly required hospitalization, to be routinely performed on a day surgery basis. There already exists a wide measure of agreement among advocates of day surgery about the range of suitable procedures.

Part A of this chapter illustrates and describes some of the most common surgical procedures undertaken routinely in day surgery units. Related anatomy and normal or altered physiology are discussed, and specific pre- and postoperative care noted, along with surgical details. Part B discusses endoscopic procedures (including minimally invasive surgery) and laser surgery.

| Part A | # Common surgical procedures undertaken in day surgery |

■ CONTENTS

INTRODUCTION

This part provides specific information on the following areas of surgical intervention:

- ophthalmic surgery
- hernia repair
- varicose vein surgery
- breast surgery
- genitourinary surgery
- gynaecological surgery
- ENT surgery
- orthopaedic surgery

OPHTHALMIC SURGERY

Patients entering the day surgery unit for eye surgery exhibit many emotions and reactions, such as hostility, anger, fear, grief and helplessness. Of prime concern to most is the success of the surgical procedure.

Patients undergoing eye surgery vary from infants with congenital conditions to geriatric patients whose conditions are a result of the aging process. The aim in the management of care is to provide a high standard of personalized nursing care for patients undergoing eye surgery, in a supportive and homely environment, and also to prepare the patient and carer for home care. General knowledge of the anatomical structure involved in an operation makes possible an understanding of the surgeon's plan of treatment and the need for specific instrumentation.

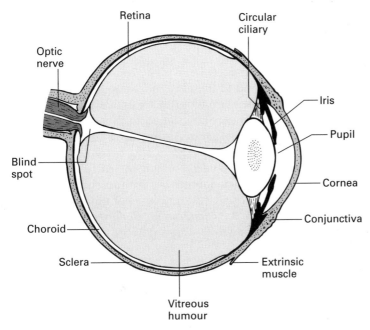

Figure 4.1 Section of the eye.

Smith (1993) states that cataract and squint surgery together account for over three quarters of all ophthalmic operations.

The eye

The eye is a complex organ that provides the sense of sight (see Figure 4.1). The eyeball has a tough outer coat called the sclera which forms the white part of the eye. The circular, most forward part of the eye is called the cornea. The cornea is transparent. Behind the cornea is a fluid-filled space called the aqueous humour (watery fluid). Moving further back, there is a black hole in its centre called the pupil. The iris changes the size of the pupil in response to changes in brightness. Directly behind the iris is the lens. The lens changes shape to help focus the light rays entering the eye, but surprisingly, most of the focusing of light rays is done by the cornea. The main body of the eye, behind the lens, is filled with a clear gel called the vitreous humour. At the very back of the eye is the retina. The light rays fall on the retina, which converts those light rays into signals that are processed by the brain, allowing us to see. The eyeball itself is moved by six delevate muscles called the ocular muscles.

Cataract

Nature, causes and treatment

What is a cataract? A cataract is a loss of transparency of the crystalline lens of the eye. A lens that is opaque to any degree is, by definition, cataractous. A cataract may or may not be significant, however, depending on how much light it scatters or blocks from entering the eye. Small lens opacities

A cataract is a loss of transparency of the crystalline lens of the eye.

are common, many being present from birth. The term cataract is generally used only to designate those opacities that impair vision. Severe cataracts are a major cause of treatable blindness.

What causes cataracts? Cataracts have many causes. Some are congenital, others develop after trauma to the eye, and some that occur in the outer layer of the lens have been linked with excessive ultraviolet radiation, as from the sun. Still others are associated with a system-wide medical problem such as diabetes. Most cataracts, however, occur as a consequence of aging. As the lens ages, it may gradually become cloudy. Spectacle changes can usually correct the vision during the early stages, but surgery may be necessary. A recent development in cataract surgery is a tiny ultrasonic probe with a tip that oscillates thousands of time per second. Placed within the eye, it can break the cataract into small pieces which are rinsed from the eye. Currently, however, these devices are not satisfactory for all patients.

How is a cataract treated? Treatment is by removal of the cloudy or opaque lens from the eye. This involves opening the eye at the edge of the cornea. The operation is performed with the aid of a microscope using careful stitching technique which enables the wound to heal correctly.

Specific preoperative preparation

On admission to the day surgery unit, a staff member should fully orient the patient to the physical surroundings. In order to familiarize the patient with the areas of the unit, it is often helpful to walk with her until she feels comfortable with her surroundings.

> Visually impaired patients should be helped to familiarize themselves with the environment of the day surgery unit. Constant reinforcement and description are important.

Constant reinforcement and description are important to the visually impaired. Consistency in nursing personnel is helpful so that the patient can recognize familiar voices and faces. In addition to routine admission information, an ocular history must also be obtained, identifying the patient's primary problem, present illness, nature of symptoms and any limitations imposed on the patient by the condition or disease. Following completion of the assessment information, including any medication the patient is taking, and identification of any patient problems, a plan of care for the entire treatment period is developed. A full blood count, chest X-ray and ECG are routinely undertaken.

Patient education

Thorough preoperative preparation plays a vital role in the successful outcome of the surgical procedure. The ophthalmic patient should be informed of the purpose and desired results of preoperative eye drops and sedation. An explanation of what to expect from the anaesthetic reduces patient anxiety levels and enables the patient to cooperate better.

A brief description of the operating room and its equipment on the patient's arrival helps to allay the patient's fears. The patient should be fully informed of what to expect immediately after surgery; reassurance is especially important for patients whose eyes will be patched postoperatively.

Operative procedure: cataract extraction with lens implant

Anaesthetic Carrie and Simpson (1988) state that local anaesthetic is preferred for most types of eye surgery. Three methods of administration are as follows: instillation of eye drops, infiltration, and block or regional anaesthetic. The infiltration method consists of an injection of anaesthetic solution beneath the skin, beneath the conjunctiva or into the tendon's capsule, depending on the type of surgery.

Block or regional anaesthetic consists of retrobulbar injection of anaesthetic solution into the base of the eyelid at the level of the orbital margin or behind the eyeball to block the ciliary ganglion and nerves. Retrobulbar injection is usually performed 10–15 minutes before surgery in order to produce temporary paralysis of the extraocular muscles.

Youth, dementia, severe anxiety, specific systemic disease and long duration of the operative procedure are among the conditions that may dictate use of general anaesthetic.

> Local anaesthetic is preferred for most types of eye surgery. Three methods of administration are: instillation of eye drops, infiltration, and block or regional anaesthetic.

Patient position, draping and cleansing of the eye The patient is transferred onto the operating table, placed in the supine position and the head placed in a Rubens pillow. The eye is cleaned using antimicrobial skin disinfectant, and drapes are carefully positioned, paying scrupulous attention to strict aseptic technique. Because many ophthalmic procedures are performed under local anaesthetic, the circulating nurse should monitor the patient and provide supportive care throughout. The theatre should be kept as quiet and peaceful as possible, to decrease the patient's anxiety.

> Aseptic technique must be scrupulously followed. The circulating nurse should monitor the patient and provide support throughout.

The scrub nurse has additional responsibilities. Foreign substances must not be introduced intraocularly. The portion of an instrument used in an intraocular wound should not be touched by the gloved hand, and all solutions used on the sterile field must be carefully labelled.

A speculum is placed in the lid to hold the lid apart; lid sutures may also be used, depending on the surgeon's preference. Endocapsular cataract extraction is one method of removing a cataract (content of the lens). A linear incision is made in the anterior capsule of the lens, the cataract is extracted through this, and an intraocular lens implant is inserted in the bag through the incision. This method ensures the intraocular lens is placed in the correct position. Once the lens is inserted, the central part of the anterior lens membrane is removed, leaving the rest of the capsular bag intact to support the lens. This type of extraction is also known as intercapsular or the 'in the bag' technique.

At the conclusion of the procedure, a combination of steroid and antibiotic solution is given subconjunctivally. The eye is padded; a plastic disposable shield is placed and taped over to protect the eye, particularly during sleep.

Specialist postoperative care

Following surgery, nursing care is planned to assist the patient to full recovery, and his or her needs and criteria for a safe discharge are assessed. At discharge, relevant verbal and written advice is given to the patient and carer, and a followup appointment is arranged. Guidelines are given as to activities which should be avoided, such as heavy lifting, stooping or rubbing the eye, for the first 2 weeks following surgery. It is advised that some discomfort is expected following surgery and paracetamol can be taken.

The day after the operation, it is essential that the patient has someone to escort him back to hospital, where the doctor will remove the eye patch and examine the eye and teach the patient or the escort how to put in eye drops.

Strabismus

> Strabismus is a misalignment of the eyes by which they focus improperly on objects and double vision results.

Strabismus is a misalignment of the eyes by which they focus improperly on objects and double vision (diplopia) occurs. Cross-eye (esotropia) involves one eye looking at an object and the other turning inward.

Children with strabismus usually subconsciously suppress the image arising from the deviating eye; eventually, this eye becomes 'lazy'. Temporary treatment consists of placing a patch over the other eye to force the use of the weak eye; but surgery may eventually be necessary to correct strabismus.

Preoperative specialist preparation

Full blood count and sickle cell test is undertaken if necessary. Informed consent is obtained from parent.

Operative procedure

Surgical approaches Two surgical approaches are used to correct strabismus: strengthening is usually accomplished by a resection procedure, and weakening is usually done with a recession procedure. Resection procedure for strabismus involves removal of a portion of ocular muscle and attachment of cut ends.

> Perioperative nurses should be aware that tension or traction on the ocular muscle can precipitate bradycardia.

Specific preparation The patient is prepared as described previously for eye surgery, and a general anaesthetic is usually used for children. Perioperative nurses should be aware that tension or traction on the ocular muscle can precipitate bradycardia.

Intraoperative procedure Supine position is used, and the child's head is positioned on a head ring. A speculum is inserted into the eye, and the conjunctiva is incised at one border of the muscle to be resected. The muscle insertion is hooked with a muscle hook, and the conjunctiva over the insertion is opened. Double ended sutures are passed through the muscle belly at the desired position of shortening, and the muscle is incised anterior to this suture. The stump of the muscle is excised from the insertion, and the muscle is then sutured to the insertion using a double ended suture. The conjunctiva is closed using an absorbable suture. At the conclusion of the procedure, antibiotic solution is given subconjunctivally, the eye is padded and a disposable shield is placed and taped over the eye.

Specialist postoperative care

Following surgery, nursing care is planned to assist the patient to a full recovery, and their needs and criteria for safe discharge are assessed. Parents are informed that their child will feel some discomfort to her eye following surgery and may therefore be rather miserable for that evening. Eye dressing may be removed before discharge from the day unit if it is found to be irritating to the child.

At discharge, relevant verbal and written advice is given to the parents, and a followup appointment is arranged. All information sheets have a 24 hour contact number and parents are advised to contact the hospital if they become concerned about the child's general condition or the area of surgery.

GENERAL SURGERY

Hernia repair

Hernia

A hernia is an abnormal protrusion of an organ or part of an organ through the structure enclosing it. The term usually refers to the protrusion of an intra-abdominal organ through the enclosing abdominal wall. It can be present at birth or it can occur when heavy strain is placed on a structurally weak point, for example where blood vessels or ducts connect with a body cavity, as in the lower abdomen. Hernias occur in the groin more frequently than in any other region (inguinal region). Congenital or indirect hernias occur due to incomplete closure of the inguinal canal following descent of the testicles in utero through the abdominal wall into the scrotum.

Hernia repair is one of the most common day surgery operations. It has been reported that in approximately forty District Health Authorities (DHAs) 10% of hernias were repaired on a day care basis. In two DHAs 40% of hernias were repaired on a day surgery basis. Nationally, up to 6% of all hernias were repaired in a day surgery setting (Audit Commission 1990).

Repair of inguinal hernia is indicated to prevent strangulation of the hernia occurring.

Inguinal hernia The inguinal canal lies in the groin and is about 4 cm long. It passes between the muscles of the anterior abdominal wall from the deep inguinal ring to the superficial inguinal ring. In the female, it contains the round ligament and in the male the spermatic cord consisting of the vas deferens and its artery, the testicular artery, the pampiniform plexus of veins, lymphatics and nerves. There are two types of inguinal hernia:

- A *direct inguinal hernia* exists when the hernial sac passes directly through the posterior wall of the inguinal canal to appear at the superficial inguinal ring, i.e. it does not transverse the inguinal canal.
- An *indirect inguinal hernia* exists when the hernial sac extends through the deep inguinal ring, the inguinal canal and the superficial inguinal ring (Figure 4.2).

Preoperative investigations

A full blood count is carried out prior to admission. If the patient is Asian,

> A hernia is an abnormal protrusion of an organ or part of an organ through the structure enclosing it – usually the protrusion of an intra-abdominal organ through the enclosing abdominal wall. Hernias occur most frequently in the groin (inguinal hernia). Hernia repair is one of the most common day surgery operations.

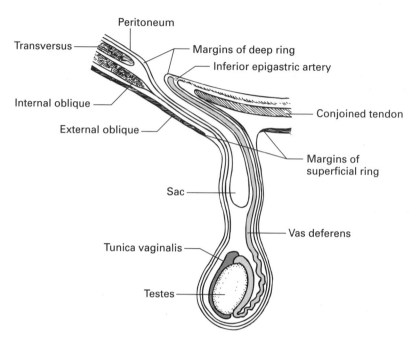

Figure 4.2 Right indirect inguinal hernia. Reproduced with permission from Ethicon 1981 Digest of Basic Surgery. Ethicon Ltd, Edinburgh.

African or Afro-Caribbean a sickle cell blood investigation is ordered. If the patient is over 50 years an ECG and chest X-ray may be carried out. Prior to admission a full preoperative nursing assessment is undertaken by a first-level nurse.

Operative procedure

Surgical approaches Repair of inguinal hernia may be performed under a local anaesthetic or a general anaesthetic. The Shouldice or Canadian operation is the most common repair undertaken (Hodge 1994). Access is gained to the hernia through a skin crease incision 2 cm above the medial half of the inguinal ligament. The external oblique aponeurosis is exposed and incised, thus opening the inguinal canal. The type of repair carried out will depend on the surgeon's preference and the extent of the hernia. To repair an indirect inguinal hernia, the spermatic cord (in men) is mobilized and retracted. The layers of the cord are separated, the sac is identified and freed to its neck at the deep inguinal ring. The sac is opened and any contents pushed back into the abdominal cavity. A transfixion suture is inserted at the neck of the sac, tied and the sac excised. Polypropylene mesh is frequently used; this is placed in the extraperitoneal space to reinforce the fascia transversalio. The mesh may be fixed with staples (Robbins & Rutrow 1993) or alternatively held in position using a 5/0 Ethilon suture.

The tissue layers are closed. Bupivacaine (Marcain 0.5%) may be infiltrated with the wound tissue to minimize postoperative pain. Skin staples may be used to approximate skin edges; a sterile airtight dressing is then applied.

Intraoperative procedure The patient walks or may be transported on a trolley to the anaesthetic room or, if appropriate, directly onto the operating table. All safety protocols are adhered to and the patient is placed in the supine position with dependent areas supported. A diathermy plate is attached to the thigh opposite the operation site. Cleansing of the operation site follows. Different units and surgeons have individual preferences for skin and operative site preparation. It is usual for the patient to have had a bath or shower on the day of operation prior to admission.

Research into the use of antiseptic preparations to be used in the preoperative bath or shower is contradictory. Leigh et al (1983) found that a single antiseptic bath eliminated the skin carriage of *Staphylococcus aureus* but did not reduce postoperative wound infection rates. Willford (1983) suggests that there is a direct relationship between wound infection and hair removal: the lowest wound infection rates are obtained where no hair was removed, and the highest when a razor was used. As a result many surgeons no longer require the patient to be shaved before arriving at the day unit.

> Surgeons' preferences on preparation of skin vary regarding the use of antiseptics in the preoperative bath or shower and regarding shaving.

A sterile field is created by placing sterile drapes in a specific position over the prepared skin to maintain the sterility of the surface.

Specialist postoperative care

The patient is transferred to the recovery area where vital signs are recorded every 15 minutes until the patient is awake. Wound site is monitored for postoperative haemorrhage. The pain relief protocol is adhered to, ensuring the patient's comfort. Antiemetics are administered as required. An appointment is made with the GP or outpatient department for removal of skin staples, 7–10 days postoperatively.

An information leaflet or booklet is provided for patients by most day surgery units following day surgery. The information will be specific for the operation performed; Box 4.1 shows an example for postoperative hernia repair.

Varicose vein surgery

Varicose veins

Varicose veins develop when blood flow in the legs becomes permanently sluggish and the veins permanently dilate. Other forms of venous varicosities are haemorrhoids and varicocele. Many factors contribute to the cause of varicose veins. The underlying cause may be a congenital weakness in the walls of the vein, an abnormal placement of the valves in the vein, or a defect of the valves. Immediate causes include severe physical strain such as that produced by long standing and lifting heavy objects. Pressure on pelvic veins from the enlargening of the uterus during pregnancy, pelvic tumours that may press on the veins, and obesity may also contribute to the development of varicose veins.

> Varicose veins develop when blood flow in the legs becomes permanently sluggish and the veins permanently dilate.

Indications for surgery When oedema and skin pigmentation (which can lead to ulceration) occur, surgery is usually advised. Sometimes veins are

■ **BOX 4.1 Information to patients after hernia repair**

Wound	Keep dry until removal of clips or sutures.
Pain	A prescription for appropriate analgesia may be given or patient may be advised to take own pain relief tablets, ie paracetemol.
Sexual activity	Return to normal sexual activity as soon as it feels comfortable
Driving	Is not advised for at least 2 weeks post surgery or until an emergency stop can be achieved.
Eating and drinking	A normal healthy diet is advised, avoiding constipation as this puts a strain on abdominal muscles.
Lifting	Avoid lifting any weight, e.g. shopping, suitcases, for at least 1 month after operation.
Return to work	Patients in sedentary work may return to work 2 weeks later; however, in heavy manual work, a longer period is needed.

The patient is advised to seek doctor's advice if any of the following occur:

• excessive bleeding
• severe pain
• increased swelling
• inflammation of wound site / raised temperature / fever.

so distended that they become unsightly and surgery may be performed for cosmetic reasons.

Preoperative specialist preparation

A full blood count is carried out. If a young woman is taking the contraceptive pill she may be advised to stop prior to surgery, as this may predispose her to a deep vein thrombosis or pulmonary embolism (Stephenson 1990).

The patient is advised by the surgeon to shave the pubic/groin region of the legs the night before surgery and to take a shower or bath prior to admission on the morning of the operation.

> A young woman taking the contraceptive pill may be advised to stop prior to surgery, as this may predispose her to a deep vein thrombosis or pulmonary embolism.

> The pubic/groin region should have been shaved the night before surgery.

Operative procedure

The patient walks or is transported on a trolley to the anaesthetic room and, following a general anaesthetic, is then transferred to the operating theatre table. All safety protocols are adhered to. The patient is placed in the supine position with both legs abducted and resting on a theatre table attachment.

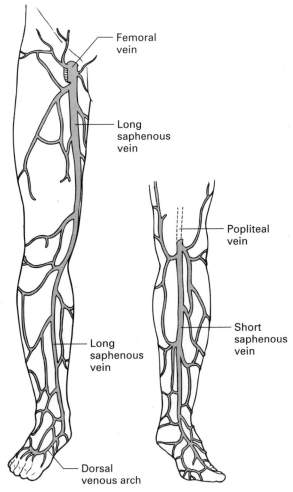

Femoral
vein

Long
saphenous
vein

Popliteal
vein

Long
saphenous
vein

Short
saphenous
vein

Dorsal
venous arch

Figure 4.3 Superficial veins of the leg. Reproduced with permission from Wilson K J W, Waugh A 1996 Anatomy and physiology in health and illness, 8th edn. Churchill Livingstone, Edinburgh.

Vein ligation and stripping Ligation and stripping is one of the most common types of surgery performed on varicose veins. As varicose veins are only prominent when the limb is dependent, the surgeon marks them out on the skin before the operation. The long saphenous vein, which branches from the groin and extends to the ankle is the one removed (See Figure 4.3). One or both legs may be involved.

The long saphenous vein is explored at its upper end through a skin crease incision. Its tributaries are secured and it is traced to its junction with the femoral vein. Here it is doubly ligated and divided. This operation alone may suffice to control varicosities, but more usually it is combined with stripping.

The vein stripper is a length of wire slightly expanded at one end and fitted with a cone-shaped head at the other. The smaller end is introduced up the long saphenous vein through a short incision in front of the medial malleolus and passed the length of the vein. Division of the vein at the ankle and tying it around the stripper allows the entire vein to be removed by pulling proximally. The groin wound is closed in layers, and the skin edges are approximated using skin clips. This is covered with an airtight dressing.

Steristrips are used to approximate the skin edges of the incision in front of the medial malleolus; this is also covered by an airtight dressing. A compression bandage is applied from ankle to groin using wool and crepe bandages.

Specialist postoperative care

The patient is transferred to recovery, where a complete handover is given to the recovery nurse. The wound sites are observed for any bleeding, and the colour, warmth and sensation are checked to ensure that the blood and nerve supplies to the limbs are intact. The patient is mobilized as soon as possible.

An information leaflet or booklet is provided, the information being specific to varicose veins (see Box 4.2). An outpatient appointment is given on discharge, as is a letter for the patient's GP giving details of the operation.

BREAST SURGERY

The breasts

The breasts, or mammary glands, lie on the anterior chest wall. The cylindrical projection on the skin surface forms the nipple, which is perforated by duct orifices. The pinkish area of skin around it is referred to as areola; this becomes pigmented during pregnancy. The breast consists of 15–20 lobes, each with a duct that opens onto the surface of the nipple. Each lobe consists of clusters of secreting cells which form lobules.

Indications for surgery

As many as one in twelve women will develop breast cancer during their lifetime.

Any abnormal lump felt in the breast is removed for diagnostic purposes. Breast cancer is a common condition affecting as many as one in every twelve women during their lifetime (Baum 1989). Like most cancers, the prognosis is greatly improved by early detection. The easiest method for enhancing early detection is breast awareness and mammography.

Through health awareness programmes women are encouraged to be breast aware and check their breasts at the same point in the menstrual cycle each month. The purpose is to note any new or unusual lumps or a change in the appearance of the breast. Unusual changes should be reported to the GP, who will refer the patient to a breast surgeon specialist (Baum 1988).

Another method for increasing early detection of breast cancer is mammography. Several studies have shown that breast cancer deaths can be decreased by routine screening of otherwise healthy women, using mammography. This should have the effect of increasing compliance within the UK Breast Cancer Screening (BSC) Programme, which is, as stated earlier, running at just over 70% (Chamberlain et al 1993). Almost 30% of women aged 50–64 years who are invited to attend the BSC pro-

■ BOX 4.2 Information to patients after varicose vein surgery.

Bandages	These should not be removed until 7–10 days post-operatively, when the clips, sutures or Steristrips are removed by the GP or outpatient department. The area should be kept dry and clean until then. Following the removal of bandages, elastic stockings are worn during the day only for 1 month. These stockings help to improve the blood circulation to the legs.
Pain	Mild pain and bruising will probably be experienced after the operation. Usual pain relief tablets should relieve the pain.
Driving	May be commenced 2 weeks after the operation or when an emergency stop can be completed successfully.
Sexual activity	May be resumed as soon as it feels comfortable.
Exercise	When resting, elevate legs, avoid putting pressure on calves.

- Do not stand for long periods
- Do not cross legs.

An exercise regime is given on the amount of daily exercise to be maintained.

Bathing	Skin must be kept clean and dry until sutures are removed. (Stephenson 1990)

Seek doctor's advice if

- severe pain is not relieved by usual pain-relieving tablets;
- the leg or groin becomes swollen;
- there is any continuous or severe bleeding;
- patient experiences fever or feels generally unwell.

gramme do not do so. These women need convincing of the benefits of screening.

Preoperative specialist investigations

Prior to surgery a full blood count is carried out. A mammogram may be ordered on women over 35 years, depending on the size, position and texture of the lump. Women over 50 years usually have a chest X-ray and electrocardiograph. Women of Asian, African and Afro-Caribbean background may require a sickle cell blood test. Ultrasound of the breast and fine needle aspiration cytology or core biopsy may be performed on palpable lesions.

Operative procedure

The patient walks or may be transported on a trolley to the anaesthetic room, where the patient's identity is ascertained and the unit's safety check protocol adhered to.

Following a general anaesthetic the patient is transferred to the operating theatre table. Again all safety protocols are adhered to, and the patient is placed in the supine position with pressure areas well supported. The appropriate arm is placed at a right angle to the body and rested on an armboard. A diathermy plate is attached to the patient's thigh.

Cleansing of the breast and the surrounding skin follows with the skin preparation of the surgeon's choice. A sterile field is created by placing sterile drapes in a specific position to maintain sterility of the surface. The incision site is then marked by the surgeon. The area of the breast may be infiltrated with bupivacaine 0.25% with adrenaline 1 : 200 000 prior to incision. The incision is made, if possible to follow the contour of the breast. The surgeon removes a minimum amount of skin to preserve the appearance of the breast. The excised lump is sent to the laboratory for analysis.

The wound may be closed using catgut on the subcutaneous layer, and the skin edges are approximated using 5/0 Dermalon. Bupivacaine 0.5% may be injected into the wound tissue prior to skin closure since this helps to control postoperative pain. A sterile airtight dressing may be applied to the wound with a pressure dressing on top.

Specific postoperative care

The patient is returned to the recovery room, where the unit's handover protocol is adhered to. The unit's pain relief protocol is implemented to ensure patient comfort. Antiemetics are administered if required.

An appointment is given to the patient to return to the breast unit or outpatient department 10 days postoperatively for removal of sutures. The histological findings from the lump are given to the patient. The following advice should be given to the patient.

- No lifting of heavy weights, stretching or carrying heavy shopping is advised.
- Avoid driving a car for 1 week.
- Avoid returning to work until the sutures have been removed.
- The wound should be kept dry until the sutures are removed.
- Mild pain relief may be needed for the first 48 hours postoperatively.
- The doctor's advice should be sought if:
  - there is continuous bleeding through dressing;
  - severe pain is not relieved by ordinary pain relief tablets;
  - there is increased swelling;
  - the patient feels generally unwell with raised temperature or fever.

Diagnosis of breast cancer can cause severe anxiety or depression. Psychological care is available both pre- and postoperatively.

Many women will develop severe anxiety or depression on discovering or being diagnosed as having a breast lesion, and if subsequently diagnosed as having cancer; this in part arises from the uncertainty of prognosis. It is vital that during the assessment phase for day surgery, the patient is given time to express fears. Psychological care is available both pre- and postoperatively.

It is helpful to have the expertise of the breast care nurse within the hospital to assess the patient's needs prior to operation and again when the patient returns to the outpatient department 1 week later (NHS Breast Screening Programme 1990).

GENITOURINARY SURGERY

Perioperative nurses involved in genitourinary surgery must have a comprehensive knowledge of the genitourinary system and special diagnostic studies and operative techniques used in this speciality.

Surgery on the male reproductive system

In the male reproductive system, sperm production begins in the innumerable seminiferous tubules within each testis. Sperm then move into the epididymis where they mature. Shortly before ejaculation, the mature sperm are propelled from the epididymis into a long tube called the 'vas deferens'. The vas deferens carries the sperm to the seminal vesicles, which add seminal fluid to the sperm cells. The semen then travels along two short ducts to the urethra. Lastly, as the semen in the urethra passes through the prostate, more secretions are added to it before it is expelled from the penis by ejaculation.

The following surgical procedures are described in detail below:

- vasectomy
- circumcision
- cystoscopy.

Vasectomy

A vasectomy is male sterilization by the surgical interruption of the vas deferens, the two sperm-transporting tubes that lead from the male testes to the ejaculatory duct. Because of the serious implications of permanent sterilization, particular attention must be paid to acquiring informed consent and counselling the patient preoperatively.

> Vasectomy is male sterilization by surgical interruption of the vas deferens. Particular attention must be paid to acquiring informed consent and counselling the patient pre-operatively.

Indications Permanent method of sterilization.

Preoperative specialist preparation

- Full blood count is carried out prior to admission if indicated.
- Informed consent is obtained.
- Counselling is given.

Intraoperative needs The patient is placed in supine position, supporting dependent areas to prevent pressure sores developing. A diathermy pad is attached to the patient's leg. The operative site is prepared with the antiseptic solution of choice and draped aseptically. The patient is kept fully informed throughout, as this procedure is performed under local anaesthetic.

> Vasectomy is performed under local anaesthetic.

Operative procedure (see Figure 4.4) The vas is identified at the neck of the scrotum, a small incision is made in the skin over the vas, and a tissue forceps is inserted into the scrotal incision to grasp the vas and deliver

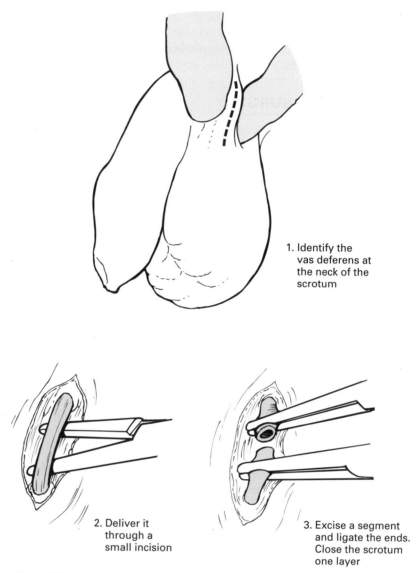

1. Identify the
vas deferens at
the neck of the
scrotum

2. Deliver it
through a
small incision

3. Excise a segment
and ligate the ends.
Close the scrotum
one layer

Figure 4.4 Vasectomy procedure. Reproduced with permission from Clark W B 1981
Digest of operative procedures. Ethicon Ltd, Edinburgh.

it to the surface. The vas is denuded of surrounding tissues, and straight
haemostats are placed at either side of the tissue forceps to crush the
vas. The vas is cut beneath the clamps. The ends of the vas deferens are
blocked either by ligation or cautery. The skin is closed using an absorbable
interrupted suture. A dressing is applied and a scrotal support is worn for
approximately seven days.

Specialist postoperative care Some discomfort and tenderness is to be
expected for a few days following surgery. Pain relief is maintained usually
by analgesics taken by the patient at home: e.g. paracetamol. Rest is necessary for 48 hours after the operation, and strenuous activity including

sexual intercourse should be avoided for 7 days. The patient wears a suspensory support for 1 week, keeping the wound dry and undisturbed. Some slight blood staining is to be expected; however, if this continues or if the dressing requires changing, the patients should contact the GP. After 7 days the suspensory support is removed and a bath can be taken.

After vasectomy the male is not sterile until sperm that has already been stored in the seminal vesicles is flushed from the system; therefore the client continues to use a method of birth control until told by the GP that semen is free from sperm. The client is given an outpatient appointment and two appointments for semen analysis postoperatively. Clients should report to their GP if:

- the incision bleeds excessively;
- they notice any pus or discharge;
- they have a temperature above 37.6°C.

Circumcision

Circumcision is the excision of the foreskin (prepuce) of the glans penis.

> Circumcision is the excision of the foreskin of the glans penis.

Indications

- relief of phimosis
- prevention of recurrent pharaphimosis
- prophylactically in infancy for religious reasons
- recurrent balanitis.

Preoperative specialist preparation A full blood count is carried out and a sickle cell test on children.

Operative procedure The client is prepared for either a local or general anaesthetic, supine position is used and routine skin preparation and draping is employed.

The dorsal surface of the foreskin is grasped with an artery forceps and gently pulled downwards until it is held on the stretch. If phimosis is severe, a second artery forceps is used as a dilator to enlarge the opening. Using a probe in the infant or an artery forceps in the adult, the foreskin is freed from the glans so that it can be completely retracted leaving no adhesions behind. The foreskin is pulled down over the glans, two straight artery forceps are placed side by side in the midline on the dorsal surface of the foreskin. An incision is made between the forceps, the incision is continued in the same direction about 3–5 mm short of the corona. Cutting laterally until the incision reaches the lateral border of the glans, the incision is carried towards the fraenum, ensuring that both surfaces of the foreskin are cut together. Bleeding vessels are coagulated or clamped with mosquito haemostats and tied with a fine catgut ligature. The raw edges of the skin incision are approximated to a coronal cuff of mucosal pruce with a fine absorbable catgut suture. Sterile lignocaine gel 0.5% is applied to the wound site postoperatively as this acts as a local anaesthetic and prevents the exposed skin adhering to the underclothes.

Specialist postoperative care Following surgery the patient is advised

The patient is advised not to take lengthy baths or showers. Complete healing will take at least 1 month. Children are usually advised to take a week off school.

that the penis will be swollen and painful for 2 or 3 days. Adult patients will be given a prescription for paracetamol or distalgesic; for infants any discomfort may be eased by Calpol syrup.

The patient is advised not to have lengthy baths or showers as this will dissolve the sutures too quickly. It will be at least 1 month before complete healing occurs. Children are usually advised to have a week off school, and, following return to school, a week off games and PT is advisable.

An appointment will be given to attend an outpatient clinic in 4–6 weeks time. Patients are advised to contact their GP should any problems arise postoperatively.

Cystoscopy

A cystoscopy is an endoscopic examination of the urinary tract.

A cystoscopy is an endoscopic examination of the urinary tract, including visual inspection of the interior of the urethra, bladder and ureteral orifice using a cystoscope, a versatile optical instrument with a variety of telescopic lenses. In male patients the verumontanum, the ejaculatory ducts, the bladder neck and the medial and lateral lobes of the prostate are examined. In female patients, the urethra, bladder neck and bladder are examined.

Indications

- diagnostic purposes
- haematuria
- urinary incontinence
- urinary tract infection
- tumour
- fistula.

Preoperative specific preparations A full blood count will be carried out, plus if necessary a chest X-ray and ECG.

The anaesthetized patient is placed in the lithotomy position on the operating table. Correct positioning of the patient is imperative to ensure optimum relaxation of leg muscles and perineum.

Operative procedure The patient is prepared for a general anaesthetic. Following anaesthetic the patient is transferred onto the operating table and placed in the lithotomy position. Correct positioning of the patient is imperative so as to ensure optimum relaxation of leg muscles and perineum, and so reduce pressure on the popliteal areas.

If the cystoscope procedure requires the use of an electrosurgical unit, the diathermy pad is placed on the patient in direct contact with the skin, as close to the operative site as practical, usually on the upper thigh.

The entire pubic area, including the scrotum and perineum, is prepped using an antimicrobial solution.

After correct positioning of the patient, the entire pubic area, including the scrotum and perineum, is cleaned using an antimicrobial solution, and the patient is draped according to surgeon's preference. When the bladder is to be opened or manipulated, a continuous flow of sterile distilled irrigation fluid is administered using a sterile closed administration set which prevents the risk of inherent cross-infection.

This allows the bladder to be distended for effective visualization. The cystourethroscope is lubricated and inserted through the urethra into the bladder. The light lead and irrigation tubing are attached to the telescope and cystoscope, and the examination is performed. Stone removal, bladder biopsy or bladder fulguration may be performed by using special cysto-scopic accessories. For retrograde urethral catheterization and pyelography, ureteral catheters are passed through the cystoscope sheath, through the ureteral orifice and into the ureter. A radio-opaque substance such as urographin 30% is then injected, and an X-ray film is taken to outline the entire upper urinary collecting system.

On completion of the procedure the patient is placed in the supine position by simultaneously removing the legs from the lithotomy position, supporting the joints above and below to prevent strain on the lumbosacral musculature.

Specialist postoperative care The patient is taken to the recovery room where he will safely recover from anaesthetic.

Some discomfort and tenderness is to be expected postoperatively. Patients are advised to maintain pain at a tolerable level by taking analgesic regularly and before the pain becomes problematic. The patient is informed that his urine may be a pink colour and that some small clots may be passed. This is a normal process following a cystoscopy, and the patient should be reassured that, as they urinate more frequently, the clotting will subside and the urine will return to its normal colour. The patient is advised to drink 2–3 litres of water per day. The patient is encouraged to do normal activities according to how they are feeling but to avoid strenuous physical activity, especially heavy lifting.

> The patient is informed that his urine may be pink and that some small clots may be passed. He is advised to drink 2–3 litres of water per day.

The patient must contact his doctor if:

- he is unable to urinate and/or feels unusual pressure within 8 hours after leaving hospital;
- he passes dark red urine and/or large blood clots;
- he is urinating very frequently (small amounts for longer than 2 days);
- he suffers from a burning sensation when urinating, which lasts more than 2 days.

Patients must complete the course of antibiotics despite feeling well. A followup appointment will be given to the patient on discharge from the day surgery unit.

GYNAECOLOGICAL SURGERY

The uterus

The uterus is a pear-shaped hollow muscular organ. It lies in the pelvic cavity in front of the rectum and behind the urinary bladder. Its position is one of anteversion and antiflexion.

The uterus measures 7.5 cm in length, 5 cm in breadth and 2.5 cm in thickness and weighs 40–50 g. It is divided into the body or fundus, the isthmus and the cervix which opens into the vagina. The uterine wall can be divided into three layers:

- an inner layer called the endometrium
- a middle layer called the myometrium
- an outer serosa or perimetrium.

The common gynaecological procedures carried out in a day surgery unit are:

- dilation and curettage
- hysteroscopy
- termination of pregnancy.

Dilation and curettage (D&C)

This is a diagnostic procedure in which the cervix is gradually dilated using graduated uterine dilators (see Figure 4.5). This allows the passage of a curette to remove a biopsy of endometrial tissue for laboratory examination.

Indications This procedure is usually performed on women who present with menorrhagia. A number of different gynaecological conditions can result in this distressing symptom. Among the most common are fibroids; these are benign tumours of the myometrium. Some fibroids may be large enough for the doctor, and sometimes the woman, to feel on palpation, or there may be many small fibroids which can be asymptomatic.

Endometriosis also causes menorrhagia; this is usually associated with pain and is quite distressing. Endometrial tissue develops outside the uterine cavity; this responds to the ovarian hormones so that at menstruation it bleeds. As this blood is incapable of escaping, it tends to form cysts; these are called chocolate cysts, named after the altered appearance of the blood.

Dysfunctional uterine bleeding is a condition in which hormonal imbalance occurs, resulting in overstimulation of the endometrium and consequent heavy bleeding.

Preoperative specialist preparation

Prior to surgery a full blood count is undertaken to detect any abnormality,

> D&C is a diagnostic procedure in which the cervix is gradually dilated using graduated uterine dilators. This allows the passage of a curette to remove a biopsy of endometrial tissue for laboratory examination. It is usually performed on women who present with menorrhagia.

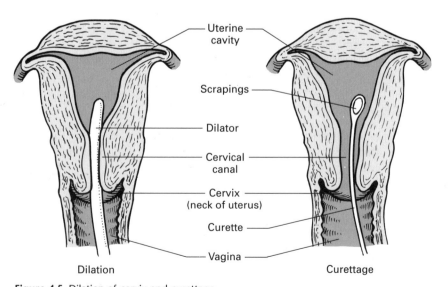

Figure 4.5 Dilation of cervix and curettage.

e.g. iron-deficiency anaemia, which will be treated appropriately prior to surgery. Gould (1985) found that many of the women interviewed described the distress and embarrassment caused by their heavy periods. A sickle cell test may also be carried out.

> A full blood count is carried out pre-operatively to detect any abnormality, e.g. iron-deficiency anaemia.

Operative procedure

The patient may walk or be transported on a trolley to the anaesthetic room. A general anaesthetic is administered. The patient is then transferred to the operating table, where the legs are placed in the lithotomy position.

> The anaesthetized patient is placed in the lithotomy position on the operating table.

Cleansing of the vulval area and vagina is carried out by the surgeon using his choice of cleansing solution. A sterile field is created by placing sterile drapes in a specific position to maintain the sterility of the surface. The patient is then catheterized to empty the bladder. The procedure is carried out as stated earlier by using graduated uterine sounds to dilate the cervix to obtain a specimen of the endometrium for laboratory investigation.

On completion of the surgical procedure the legs are simultaneously removed from the stirrups, and a sanitary towel is placed over the vagina. The patient is transferred to the appropriate recovery area. A complete report on the status of the patient, procedure performed, medication administered, dressing and allergies, is communicated to the recovery nurse by the intraoperative nurse with the appropriate documentation.

Specialist postoperative care

The patient is transferred to the recovery area where vital signs are recorded quarter hourly until the patient is awake.

An information leaflet or booklet is provided for patients following day surgery by most day surgery units. The information will be specific for the operation performed, e.g. for D&C:

- Vaginal bleeding may continue for up to 2 weeks. However, if this is heavy, e.g. soaking of a sanitary towel every 1–2 hours, the patient is advised to consult the GP or return to hospital.
- Pain – some cramping pains may be experienced for a few hours following surgery; these may be similar to period pains. The patient is advised to rest for the remainder of the day and take paracetamol if required.
- Sexual activity – return to normal sexual activity as soon as it feels comfortable and bleeding has subsided.
- Patient is advised to shower rather than have a bath, for 3 days postoperatively.
- Return to work – patients in sedentary work may return to work 2 days postoperatively, however, if in heavy work, a longer period of time off work may be necessary.

Hysteroscopy

A hysteroscopy is an examination of the uterus using a hysteroscope, which is an instrument with a fibre optic light.

The indications are those for a D&C, and the same procedure is followed.

> A hysteroscopy is an examination of the uterus using a hysteroscope, which is an instrument with a fibre optic light.

The difference is that, instead of passing a curette through the dilated cervix, a hysteroscope is passed into the uterus. A litre of normal saline is placed in a pressure cuff for irrigation of the uterine cavity. This procedure is very similar to a cystoscopy. A camera may be attached to the hysteroscope, which allows for magnification of the endometrium; this may help with diagnosis.

Intraoperative and postoperative care is the same as that for a D&C.

Therapeutic termination of pregnancy

Preparation of the patient is as for a D&C, with emphasis on the psychological care and counselling undertaken during the assessment phase.

Specialist postoperative care

Patient is discharged following a routine gynaecological procedure approximately 4 hours after the operation, into the care of a responsible adult.

The patient is given an information leaflet or booklet regarding the amount of vaginal bleeding to expect and the procedure to follow if haemorrhaging should occur, or symptoms of pyrexia above 37.6°C.

Abdominal cramps may occur as a result of those procedures; appropriate pain relief is prescribed to be taken by the patient at home, e.g. paracetamol. Normal sexual activity may resume when the patient feels comfortable to do so. If the patient is in sedentary work, e.g. office work, she may return to work 3–4 days following the procedure, but for those in heavy occupations a longer period off work is advised.

EAR, NOSE & THROAT SURGERY

There are a large number of minor procedures in ENT surgery that can be readily managed on a day surgery basis. Day surgery has a number of attractions in the field of paediatric care one being that of reduced cost. White (1992) stated that there is a wealth of research demonstrating the far-reaching psychological consequences of hospitalization of young children. Ellerton & Craig (1994) and Muller & Harris (1992) further suggest that children under 5 years of age are particularly susceptible to the detrimental effects of hospitalization.

> Nurses must bear in mind that otological surgery patients have a significant hearing loss and require additional time when procedures are described to them.

The preoperative assessment of the patient or child undergoing otological surgery should include all elements of an assessment done for any other type of surgery. The nurse must bear in mind that these patients have a significant hearing loss and require additional time when procedures are described to them.

Myringotomy

> A myringotomy is an incision of the tympanic membrane to allow drainage of pus.

A myringotomy is an incision of the tympanic membrane to allow drainage of pus. It is indicated by acute otitis media.

Preoperative specialist preparation

Full blood count and sickle cell test. Hearing test.

Operative procedure

This procedure is performed under general anaesthetic. The use of a topical analgesic cream on the dorsum of the hand, placed by the admission nurse over a suitable vein, has made venepuncture more acceptable to many small children.

The child is placed in the supine position. The ear is prepared and draped according to surgeon's preference. With microscopic visualization the aural speculum is inserted in the ear canal (see Figure 4.6). The excess cerumen is removed with a forceps. Using a sharp myringotomy knife a small curved incision is made in the anterior inferior quadrant of the pars tensa, and the membrane is cut.

A culture swab may be taken to determine the type of organism present. Pus and fluid are suctioned from the middle ear. A tube (grommet) may be inserted into the incision using an alligator forceps to allow ventilation of the middle ear. There are many different types of disposable myringotomy tubes (grommets) available for implantation, and the choice depends on the length of time the surgeon wishes the tube to remain in place. Once the tube falls out, the tympanic membrane incision usually heals. Antibiotic drops may be instilled following the insertion of the grommets.

> In the administration of general anaesthetic, the use of a topical analgesic cream on the dorsum of the hand, placed by the admission nurse over a suitable vein, has made venepuncture more acceptable to many small children.

Special postoperative care – discharge and followup

Hall (1989) states that myringotomy is associated with minimal pain postoperatively. Some children may complain of mild earache; this can be treated with paracetamol elixir (Calpol). Parents are advised that there may be a little fluid or even blood oozing from the ears in the immediate post-

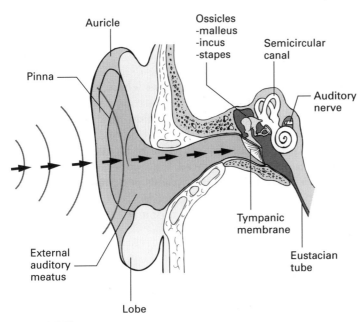

Figure 4.6 The ear.

operative period. This is a normal process, but if it persists the GP should be contacted. Children who just have grommets inserted may return to school 1 or 2 days after their operation. Parents are advised that children should avoid getting water in the ears which may introduce infection. Cotton wool can be placed in the ear canal when washing the hair or having a bath. Swimming is allowed, but wearing ear plugs and a swimming hat are important precautions. A date and time for a followup appointment within 2 weeks is given to the parents.

Realignment of a nasal fracture

Repair of nasal fracture involves manipulation and mobilization of nasal bones. If the nose has been struck by a direct frontal blow, both nasal bones are usually fractured, displaced outwards and depressed into the ethmoidal sinus. The septal cartilage is usually broken or deviated and the lateral cartilage is displaced.

Preoperative specialized preparation

Full blood count and X-ray of nose and skull.

Operative procedure

> Nasal fracture repair is considered a clean procedure, and the patient is usually neither draped nor prepped. After manipulation of the nasal bones, a plaster of Paris splint is usually applied and left in situ for approximately 1 week.

This procedure is usually performed under general anaesthetic. The patient is safely transferred onto the operating table and placed in the supine position. It is considered a clean procedure, and the patient is usually neither draped nor prepped. The surgeon wears sterile gloves and uses a rubber-shod narrow forceps or Asch septum-straightening forceps, which is inserted into the nostril. The nasal bones are elevated and moulded into place by external manipulation. A plaster of Paris splint is usually applied and left in situ for approximately 1 week.

Specialist postoperative care

> If, after discharge, the nose bleeds persistently, the patient should attend the casualty department immediately.

The patient is taken to the recovery room where he is safely recovered. The patient is put in the upright position as soon as he has recovered from anaesthetic, is breathing spontaneously and shows vital signs within normal limits. On discharge the patient is advised to take paracetamol for pain relief as prescribed. His nose may be blocked for a few days, and some blood clots are to be expected. The patient is encouraged not to blow his nose for 2–3 days. If the nose bleeds persistently the patient should attend the casualty department immediately.

The patient is given an outpatient appointment to return in 1 week to have the plaster of Paris removed.

ORTHOPAEDIC SURGERY

Orthopaedic surgery has been defined by the American Academy of Orthopaedic Surgeons as *'the medical speciality that includes the investigation, pre-*

servation, restoration and development of the form and function of the extremity, spine and associated structures by medical, surgical and physical method'. The nurse's role in patient selection and preparation involves:

- accurate assessment of the patient
- preparation of patient for surgical procedure
- effective pain control
- preparing the patient and carers for self-care at home.

The following operative procedures will be discussed in detail:

- arthroscopy of the knee
- arthroscopic menisectomy
- Dupuytren's contracture
- hallux valgus
- carpal tunnel decompression.

Arthroscopy of the knee

An arthroscopy is an endoscopic procedure which permits inspection and exploration (Jackson 1986). Arthroscopic examination of the knee joint was first performed by Professor K Tagaki in 1918. Arthroscopy is now routinely used in the diagnosis of knee joint injuries and disorders and as a prelude to endoscopic procedures, providing the surgeon with an accurate intra-articular assessment without the risk of open arthrotomy.

> An arthroscopy is an endoscopic procedure which permits inspection and exploration.

The knee

The knee is the hinge joint that connects the main bones of the leg (the femur and the tibia). The kneecap (patella) lies over the front of the joint. There are strong ligaments on both sides of the joint called the medial and lateral collateral ligaments. There are also two ligaments within the joint, called the anterior and posterior cruciate ligaments. All four of these ligaments serve to connect the bones of the knee and to provide additional stability. Like other moveable joints, the bony ends of the femur and tibia are separated by protective cartilage which serves as a cushion between the bones. There are two of these cartilage cushions in the knee. They are called medial and lateral menisci.

The powerful quadriceps muscles are responsible for straightening (extending) the leg at the knee joint. These muscles are in the front of the thigh. The kneecap is actually a large bone within the quadriceps tendon. The quadriceps tendon is thus commonly referred to as the patellar tendon. The hamstrings are the muscles which bend (flex) the knee at the knee joint. These muscles are located in the back of the thigh.

There are a number of common knee injuries. Severe twisting of the knee will frequently sprain one of the knee ligaments. A sprain and a strain are often confused. A sprain occurs when a ligament (fibrous connection between bones) is damaged. A strain occurs when a muscle or tendon is damaged. Running can sometime injure the knee by straining the patellar tendon. The cartilage cushions (menisci) within the knee are also frequently damaged by severe twisting. A torn meniscus is very painful and usually requires surgical repair.

Indications

Indications for arthroscopy are:

- confirmation of suspected meniscule lesion;
- assessment of anterior cruciate ligament integrity;
- localization of loose bodies;
- diagnosis of inflammatory joint disease and synovial biopsy;
- excision of fat pad, division of adhesions and lateral release of extension mechanism;
- diagnosis and assessment of osteoarthritis.

Arthroscopy and day surgery

Improved surgical techniques and modern anaesthetics permit arthroscopy to be performed safely as a day case procedure.

Anaesthetic technique General anaesthetic is the preferred method in the majority of cases. It allows for the comfortable use of a tourniquet, avoids the need for multiple injections of local anaesthetic, and the knee joint can be readily unlocked or manipulated for the purpose of improving the surgeon's view.

Specific preoperative preparation

Weight, blood pressure and urinanalysis are recorded on all patients undergoing general anaesthetic (Ogg 1985). A haemoglobin test is performed in all adults and those with symptoms/signs of anaemia. Sickle screen is required where appropriate, i.e. in all African and Caribbean patients, and in Greek, Turkish, Middle Eastern and Indian patients with a family history of sickle disease. Urea and electrolyte tests are performed if patients are on therapy known to cause abnormalities (e.g. diuretics). ECG is required in patients over 50 and where there is a history of hypertension or cardiovascular problems.

Operative procedure

After administration of general anaesthetic, a high-thigh pneumatic tourniquet is applied to the leg, and the leg is exsanguinated.

The patient is safely transferred to the anaesthetic room. The patient's vital signs are monitored by use of electrocardiogram (ECG), pulse oximetry, non-invasive blood pressure monitor and general observation. The nurse/ODA assists the anaesthetist and general anaesthetic is administered. The tourniquet is then applied around the thigh to restrict blood flow to the area and to ensure unhampered visualization. There are many factors to be considered when applying a tourniquet. Some of these include: the site of the cuff, method of exsanguination, the pressure of the cuff and the duration of tourniquet time. The skin directly below the cuff should be protected with orthopaedic wool: the correct size cuff should always be used.

A high-thigh pneumatic tourniquet is applied to the leg. The leg is exsanguinated. Phillips (1991) states that it is generally accepted that the pressure applied should always be related to the patient's blood pressure, as recorded following induction of anaesthetic. When using a tourniquet on the upper limb, pressure should be no more than 50 mmHg above the patient's systolic pressure, and the lower limb pressure should be twice the systolic blood pressure provided the patient is not unduly muscular or obese. There are still no clear-cut rules as to a safe time limit for the duration of tourniquet inflation. It is generally accepted, however, that a time of 2 hours is safe. If this time is exceeded, the surgeon is informed and the tourniquet may be deflated hourly. Safety does not depend on time alone, but also upon the pressure of the cuff and the adequacy of soft tissue mass.

Following application of tourniquet the patient is safely transferred onto the operating table and placed in supine position. The limb is surgically prepared according to surgeon's preference; the sterile field is created by placement of sterile drapes in a specific position to maintain sterility of the surface on which sterile instrumentation and gloved hands may be placed.

Operative technique The anterolateral approach is the most useful for routine arthroscopic examination of the knee. With the knee flexed to 90°, using a size 10 blade, a 5 mm transverse stab incision, 5 mm above the lateral tibial condule (to avoid the lateral meniscus) and 5 mm lateral to the patellar tendon is made in the skin and extended down through the joint capsule (see Figure 4.7).

The arthroscopic sheath is inserted into the joint; once settled inside the joint the trocar is removed and replaced by the telescope, which is locked into the sheath. The light cable and video systems are attached and the distension and irrigation systems assembled. Distension of the joint is achieved by a closed administration 'sterile set' connected from a litre bag of normal saline (suspended 1 metre above the knee) to the inlet tap on the arthroscope sheath. A drainage tube is connected to the outlet tap of the arthroscope and led to a bowl beneath the table. A second stab incision is made on the opposite side of the joint to allow inspection of all compartments. This also provides an entry for other arthoscopic instruments required, such as a probe, rongeur, grabber, biopsy forceps blade, cutter or curette.

The knee is manoeuvred by the surgeon, enabling internal examination of the whole joint. The joint is irrigated copiously at the end of the procedure until clear of blood and any particles. Fluid is then expressed from the joint, at the end of the procedure, down the empty sheath, which is then withdrawn completely.

Bupivacaine (Marcain) 0.25% may be injected intra-articularly to minimize postoperative pain.

The skin portals are closed using sterile skin 'steri-strips' or fine microfilament nylon sutures. A sterile dressing is applied, and the knee is supported with a compression bandage of wool and crepe extending from the tibial tuberosity to the lower leg. The tourniquet is removed and the patient is transferred to the recovery room.

Specialist postoperative care

The patient is safely recovered from anaesthetic, and a check is made on the neurovascular status of the limb. To ensure that the nerve and blood

When using a tourniquet on the upper limb, pressure should be no more than 50 mmHg above the patient's systolic blood pressure, and the lower limb pressure should be twice the systolic pressure provided the patient is not unduly muscular or obese. Although there are no clear-cut rules as to a safe time limit for the duration of tourniquet inflation, it is generally accepted that 2 h is safe. If this time is exceeded, the surgeon should be informed and the tourniquet may be deflated hourly.

The knee is supported with a compression bandage of wool and crepe extending from the tibial tuberosity to the lower leg.

Postoperatively, the nurse will check colour, sensation and movement of the distal part of the limb and will check the limb for pulses. Haemarthrosis is a relatively common complication following arthroscopic surgical procedure. If this happens, the knee will be very painful, and it will be impossible to lift the foot off the bed. A large haemarthrosis should always be aspirated.

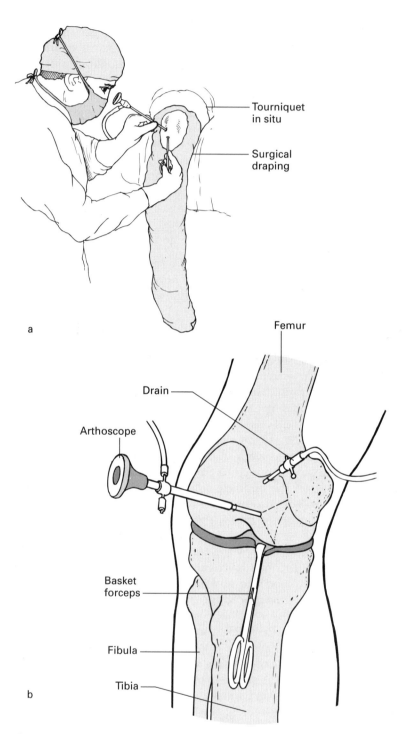

Tourniquet in situ

Surgical draping

a

Femur

Drain

Arthoscope

Basket forceps

Fibula

Tibia

b

Figure 4.7 Arthroscopy of the knee: (A) general approach; (B) detail.

supply are functioning fully, the nurse will check colour, sensation and movement of the distal part and will check the limb for pulses. Jackson (1986) and Stother (1984) state that haemarthrosis is a relatively common complication following arthroscopic surgical procedure such as lateral release. If this happens, the knee will be tender, very painful, and it will be absolutely impossible to lift the foot off the bed. A large haemarthrosis should always be aspirated.

If sutures are used, an appointment with the outpatient clinic or with the GP will be required. Sutures are usually removed after 7–10 days.

Straight-leg raising should commence immediately postoperatively, and flexion and weight-bearing should begin within 24 hours, following reduction of the compression dressing. Most patients can walk comfortably the day after the operation, although with a slight limp. Patients with light occupation such as office work can usually return to work within 1 week, but those in heavy occupations may need 2 or more weeks off. Patients should report symptoms of temperature above 37.5°C, redness, numbness (after 24 hours), tingling or any excessive drainage.

> Straight-leg raising should commence immediately postoperatively, and flexion and weight-bearing should begin within 24 h, following reduction of the compression dressing.

Arthroscopic surgical procedures

Menisectomy

The range of arthroscopic surgical procedures is continually increasing. A tear in the meniscus is the most common injury of the knee requiring surgery. It is almost always caused by acute rotation strain, usually during sporting activities, and the two classical symptoms of this condition are locking of the joint and giving way of the joint.

> A tear in the meniscus is the most common injury of the knee requiring surgery.

Indications for surgery Tear in the meniscus.

Preparation of patient As for arthroscopy.

Operative technique Arthroscopic examination of the knee is necessary to confirm diagnosis. It is possible to remove the offending meniscus arthroscopically using arthroscopic instrumentation such as scissors, blades, grabbers and biopsy forceps.

Wound closure As for arthroscopy.

Specialist postoperative care A large compression bandage is applied to support the joint. The patient may be allowed to bear weight fully on the limb or to be partially weight bearing with crutches. Patients are encouraged to attend knee classes until full strength in the joint is regained. Sutures are removed after 7–10 days. The postoperative care regimes following arthroscopy and arthroscopic menisectomy are similar.

Hand surgery

Dupuytren's contracture

This is produced by progressive thickening and contractions of the palmar aponeurosis. This results in inflection of the ring, little and middle finger in severe cases. The surgical procedure includes fasciotomy (simple division of contracted bands) or partial or total excision of the palmar fascia.

> Dupuytren's contracture is produced by progressive thickening and contractions of the palmar aponeurosis of the hand.

A tourniquet is applied around the arm to restrict blood flow and to ensure unhampered visualization.

Specific preoperative preparation A blood count, ECG and CXR, depending on age and medical history, are taken. X-ray of hand, and sickle cell test if appropriate, are taken.

Operative procedure The patient is prepared for either a local or general anaesthetic as specified. The patient is placed in the supine position on the operating table with the arm extended on the arm table. A tourniquet is applied around the arm to restrict blood flow and to ensure unhampered visualization.

The incision lines are marked, often with Z-plasties to lengthen the involved skin of the fingers and palm, (see Figure 4.8). After incisions are made, flaps of skin and subcutaneous tissues are carefully elevated to preserve their blood supply, exposing the fibrotic palmar fascia and its digital extensions. Part or all of the palmar fascia and digital extensions are excised.

The tourniquet is usually deflated before the skin is closed, to ensure that all bleeding points are secure. The incisions are sutured using a fine microfilament nylon suture. Copious dressings of soft gauze are then applied over the palm and around the affected fingers, which are held semiflexed.

Postoperative care *Wound closure:* non-absorbable sutures such as Ethilon 3/0 are usually used and will require removal after 2 weeks. An appointment for the outpatient clinic will be necessary.

The hand is kept elevated for approximately 48 hours. Early proximal interphalangeal motion is encouraged, and the shoulder is moved actively at intervals to avoid cramping.

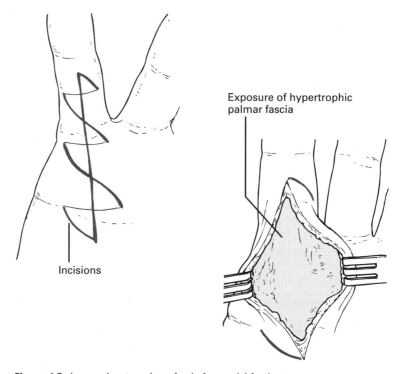

Incisions

Exposure of hypertrophic palmar fascia

Figure 4.8 Approaches to palmar fascia for partial fasciectomy.

Patients should report symptoms of temperature above 37.6°C or undue pain in the hand, as this may indicate the formation of a haematoma which should be evacuated immediately. Otherwise, the first dressing is removed after 1 week; the hand is redressed and splinted at the wrist for another week. During this second week, with the wrist still splinted, the patient is encouraged to move all the finger joints. Following removal of sutures after 2 weeks the hand is left free of all dressing. Moderate use of the hand is permitted at 3 weeks; however, several months of rehabilitation may be necessary.

Carpal tunnel release

Carpal tunnel syndrome Carpal tunnel syndrome is an entrapment process in which the median nerve (see Figure 4.9) becomes compressed at the volar surface of the wrist because of thickened synovium, trauma or aberrant muscle.

Indications for surgery Pain, numbness and tingling of the fingers. Weakness of the intrinsic thumb muscles.

Preoperative specific preparation Full blood count, sickle cell test if necessary, and X-ray of hand are taken.

> The hand is kept elevated for approximately 48 h. Patients should report high temperature or undue pain in the hand, as this may indicate the formation of a haematoma which should be evacuated immediately. Otherwise the first dressing is removed after 1 week; the hand is redressed and splinted at the wrist for another week.

> Carpal tunnel syndrome is an entrapment process in which the median nerve becomes compressed at the volar surface of the wrist.

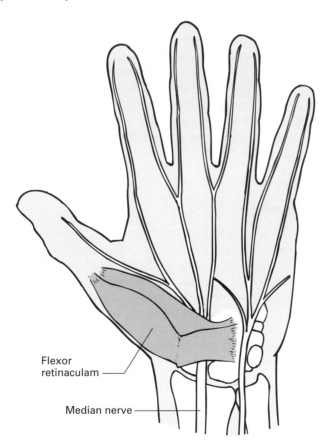

Flexor retinaculam

Median nerve

Figure 4.9 Median nerve in the hand.

Operative procedure This procedure can be performed under local, axillary block or general anaesthetic. General anaesthetic is the preferred method; it has advantages for both the surgeon and the patient, it allows for the comfortable use of a tourniquet and avoids the need for multiple injections of local anaesthetic.

> A pneumatic tourniquet is inflated around the arm.

The patient is placed in the supine position on the operating table with the arm extended on a hand table. A pneumatic tourniquet is inflated, the skin is cleaned and the limb is draped according to surgeon's preference.

After appropriate skin marking, the fingers and thumb may be controlled by a 'lead hand'. The incision is made across the volar wrist surface and the base of the palm for adequate exposure of the transverse carpal ligament. The transverse carpal ligament is incised along its entire length. A segment of it may be excised. Synovectomy of the structure within the carpal canal may or may not be performed. After release of the tourniquet and ligature of any persistent bleeding points, the skin is closed with fine monofilament suture. A compression dressing and a volar splint are applied, and the patient is transferred to the recovery room.

Specific postoperative care *Wound care:* non-absorbable sutures such as Ethilon 3/0 are usually used; these will require removal. An appointment with the outpatient clinic or with the GP will be given to the patient. Sutures are usually removed 10–14 days postoperatively.

Pain: some degree of pain is to be expected following this procedure. Pain relief is maintained usually by analgesic taken by the patient at home.

> The hand is actively used as soon as possible after surgery. The compression dressing is removed after 1 week, and a small airstrip dressing is applied. The patient is encouraged to wear a splint for 14–21 days.

Mobilization: the hand is actively used as soon as possible after surgery. The compression dressing is removed after 1 week, and a small airstrip dressing is applied. The patient is encouraged to wear a splint for 14–21 days. The patient is encouraged to seek advice if any of the following occurs: continuous bleeding, severe pain, increased swelling, coldness or numbness of fingers, change in normal colour of the fingers, or feeling generally unwell with a fever.

Foot surgery

Hallux valgus surgery

> Hallux valgus is a condition in which the big toe is deviated laterally at the metatarso-phalangeal joint.

Hallux valgus This is a condition in which the big toe is deviated laterally at the metatarso-phalangeal joint. Symptoms include pain on the dorso-medial aspect of the first metatarsal head or directly over the medial exostosis, swelling of the big toe, painful plantar callus and discomfort to the entire foot as the forefoot in general becomes more fatigued and symptomatic, with pain radiating to the leg and knee.

Hallux valgus is treated with a variety of surgical procedures (Kellers, McBrides, Lapidus and Mayo). All these procedures remove the exostosis and attempt to realign the big toe by removal of bone, transfer of tendons, osteotomy of the first metatarsal shaft or appropriate imbrication of soft tissue. The overall aim of surgery is to correct deformity, resection of the abnormal bony component and allow normal or near normal range of motion.

Preoperative specialist preparation Full blood count is undertaken; chest

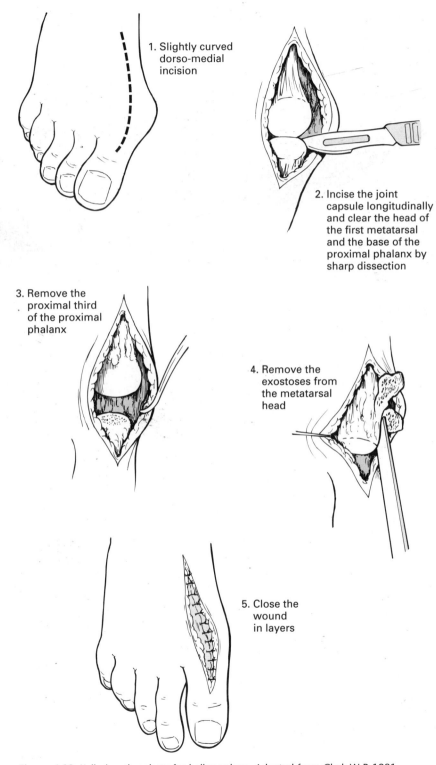

1. Slightly curved dorso-medial incision

2. Incise the joint capsule longitudinally and clear the head of the first metatarsal and the base of the proximal phalanx by sharp dissection

3. Remove the proximal third of the proximal phalanx

4. Remove the exostoses from the metatarsal head

5. Close the wound in layers

Figure 4.10 Keller's arthroplasty for hallux valgus. Adapted from Clark W B 1981 Digest of operative procedures. Ethicon Ltd, Edinburgh.

X-ray and ECG may be required depending on the patient's age and physical condition. X-ray of the foot will also be performed. Sickle cell test if necessary.

Operative procedure (see Figure 4.10) Supine position is used and the patient is prepared for local or general anaesthetic as specified. A tourniquet is applied to the proximal thigh. The foot and leg are prepared and draped according to surgeon's preference.

> A tourniquet is applied to the proximal thigh.

A slightly curved dorso-medial incision is made, the joint capsule is incised longitudinally and the head of the first metatarsal cleared, and the base of the proximal phalanx by sharp dissection. The proximal third of the proximal phalanx is removed, the exostoses from the metatarsal head is also excised. The wound is closed in layers and a soft bulky pressure dressing applied with the big toe held in the desired position. Tourniquet is removed, and the patient is transferred to the recovery room.

Specific postoperative care The foot/leg is kept elevated on a stool when resting, and the patient is encouraged to gently move her toes. Plaster of Paris is usually applied to hold the big toe in slight overcorrection and is left usually for 6 weeks. The plaster takes 24 hours to dry fully and a further 24 hours to harden. The patient is advised to rest the plaster on a pillow for the first 2 days to prevent it becoming dented. The patient can mobilize with the aid of crutches but should avoid putting weight or strain on the wound site until stitches are removed: this is usually 10 days postoperatively. The patient is advised, if toes swell or plaster feels tight around the ankle, to rest on the bed with the limb elevated for a few hours. The patient is told to keep plaster dry at all times and contact the hospital if it should become wet. The patient is also advised to contact the hospital immediately if toes swell or become blue or white or if it is difficult or painful to move. If the patient feels a sore place developing under the plaster he is advised to contact the hospital immediately.

> Plaster of Paris is usually applied to hold the big toe in slight over-correction and is left usually for 6 weeks.

Pain may be quite severe following surgery; therefore it is important that adequate analgesic is given to the patient on discharge. The patient is usually given an information sheet on discharge indicating a list of exercises to be carried out routinely.

REFERENCES

Audit Commission 1990 A short cut to better service. HMSO, London
Audit Commission 1991 Measuring quality: the patients' view of day surgery. HMSO, London
Baum M 1989 Breast cancer: the facts. Oxford University Press, New York
Carrie L E, Simpson P J 1988 Understanding anaesthesia. Heinemann, London
Chamberlain J, Moss S M, Kirkpatrick A E 1993 National Health Service Breast Screening Programme: results from 1991–1992. British Medical Journal 307: 353–356
Department of Health 1992 The health of the nation. HMSO, London
Ellerton M L, Craig M 1994 Preparing children and families psychologically for day surgery. Journal of Advanced Surgery 19: 1057–1062
Gould D G 1985 The myth of the menopause. Nursing Mirror 160(23): 25–27
Hall P 1989 In: Bradshaw E G, Davenport H T (eds) Day care: surgery, anaesthetics and management. Edward Arnold, London
Hodge D J 1994 Day surgery – hernias. Surgical Nurse 7: 4
Hutching P 1995 Advances in anaesthesia. British Journal of Theatre Nursing, 5(1)

Jackson R W 1986 The scope of arthroscopy. Clinical Orthopaedics 108: 67–71

Leigh D A 1983 Total body bathing with 'Hibiscrub' for surgical patients. Journal of Hospital Infection 4(3): 229–235

Muller D J, Harris P J 1992 Nursing children psychology: research and practice. Chapman and Hall, London

NHS Breast Screening Programme 1990 Breast cancer screening. Evidence and experience since the Forrest Report. NHSBSP, Oxford

Ogg T W 1985 Aspects of day surgery and anaesthesia. Anaesth. Rounds 18: 1–28

Phillips S 1991 Tourniquets. British Journal of Theatre Nurses (May): 13–17

Royal College of Surgeons of England 1992 Guidelines for day care surgery. Royal College of Surgeons, London

Robbins A W, Rutrow I M 1993 The mesh play hernioplasty. Surgeries of North America 73(3): 507–512

Smith H 1993 Day-release cataracts. Nursing Times 89(39): 30–33

Stother I G 1984 Arthroscopic removal of loose bodies from the knee. Journal of Royal College of Surgeons, Edinburgh 29(4): 246–248

Stephenson M E 1990 Discharge criteria in day surgery. Journal of Advanced Nursing 15: 601–613

West B 1995 Day surgery: cheaper option or challenge to care. British Journal of Theatre Nurses (April): 5–8

Wilson M 1992 Surgical nursing. Baillière Tindall, London

White A 1992 Paediatric day surgery. Nursing Times 88(39): 43–45

Willford P S 1983 Hair removal – shave, preps, depilation and other pre-operative considerations – are they really necessary? Journal of Operating Room Research Institute 3(3): 26–28

Part B

Endoscopic or laser procedures undertaken in day surgery

■ CONTENTS

A wishful dream of mankind to take a look into the darkness of the body's cavity to diagnose disease has been fulfilled for all areas of endoscopy of body cavities, thanks to the technical development of the instruments necessary. (Kurt Semm 1984)

INTRODUCTION

Special preparation needs to be considered when dealing with certain procedures within a theatre or endoscopy room environment. These are associated with minimally invasive techniques which are becoming increasingly popular within many day surgery and endoscopy departments. Many day surgery units now have their own endoscopy area, and a growing number also have their own dedicated theatre suite. Therefore an increasing number of day surgery nurses/operating department practitioners (ODPs) are maintaining and handling complicated technical equipment associated with minimally invasive surgery (MIS).

The term 'minimally invasive therapy', coined by Wickham (1991), refers to all those less invasive or non-invasive procedures that have been developed as an alternative to open surgery. As this gives the impression that no incision is required, 'minimal access surgery' is a more accurate term and is used in some circles (Hirsch & Hailey 1993). MIS has allowed more opportunities for day surgery, particularly as a result of demand from patients because of the claims of less pain, less disfigurement and a much quicker return to normal activities (Hall 1994)

All 'looking into' procedures are called endoscopy, 'endo' meaning orifice or hole and 'scopy' meaning examination. It refers to an optical instrument that carries light to illuminate and view parts of the body which are inaccessible or difficult to see by direct viewing. The optical principles and basic features of these different instruments are similar, but they can be split into two types: rigid and flexible. Generally, 'endoscopy' is used to mean flexible, though this term is actually badly used. Generalization can also be made in that flexible endoscopy is often performed under local anaesthetic or with sedation, whereas rigid endoscopy usually requires general anaesthetic.

> An endoscope is an optical instrument that carries light to illuminate and view parts of the body which are inaccessible or difficult to see by direct viewing. There are two main types: rigid and flexible. Flexible endoscopy is often performed under local anaesthetic or with sedation, whereas rigid endoscopy usually requires general anaesthetic.

Advances in technology have allowed the laser to be introduced as an option during surgery for certain techniques, either in conjunction with minimally invasive techniques or by themselves. Although not the most popular item required for the day surgery unit, such technology is becoming more popular as its benefits become more widely known.

The role of the nurse/ODP in these procedures tends to relate to health and safety and infection-control as s/he oversees storage, maintenance and usage of the equipment required for these procedures. S/he also should act as patient's advocate and support throughout the procedure.

RIGID ENDOSCOPY

Brief overview of procedures

Rigid endoscopy has been an integral part of day surgery units for many years. Procedures such as cystoscopy, arthroscopy, hysteroscopy and laparoscopy often make up a large proportion of cases within day surgery units.

Many of these procedures were purely diagnostic, with patients then having to come back at a later date for more detailed surgery on an inpatient basis. With the development of instrumentation to accompany the rigid scopes, endoscopy procedures performed in day surgery have moved away from a purely diagnostic role. This has improved the quality of service given to the patient, as now wherever possible they do not need to return for a second anaesthetic with the accompanying anxiety and inconvenience this causes.

Although this is improving the quality of service to the patient, it is also increasing the workload of the day surgery theatre or endoscopy suite team. Efficiency, speed, technical knowledge and organizational qualities are needed by the personnel working in this environment because of the special equipment and surgery rigid endoscopy requires. Originally, rigid endoscopy work was possibly viewed by staff as rather mundane since, once the procedure was underway, there was not much to see. Since the advent of the TV video chip in 1986 (Hall 1994, Greengrass & Cunningham 1995), which allowed the image from the scope to be viewed on a monitor/ screen, the pathophysiology and surgery being performed has been opened up to the rest of the surgical team. This has allowed the nurse/ODP to have a greater understanding of the procedure and means that s/he can better anticipate developments during the operation. Therefore, although technology has increased workload, it has also brought greater interest and satisfaction for supporting nurses/ODPs during these procedures.

Although rigid endoscopy is rapidly diversifying, for the purpose of this chapter only the most common procedures performed in the day surgery environment will be discussed.

Clinical conditions

The most common clinical conditions which present in day surgery for rigid scope procedures can generally be divided into three areas: gynaecological, orthopaedic and urological.

Gynaecological conditions. The anatomy of the female body is such that rigid endoscopy procedures are well suited to diagnosing and treating certain gynaecological conditions. Conditions requiring laparoscopy include:

- pelvic pain of unknown cause
- pelvic inflammatory disease (PID), often caused by chlamydia
- primary or secondary infertility
- endometriosis.

Gynaecological conditions linked to the uterus can also be viewed by hysteroscope; these include:

- intramenstrual bleeding of unknown origin
- abnormal ultrasound scan
- dysmenorrhoea
- amenorrhoea of unknown origin.

Hysteroscopy is often used to accompany dilatation and curettage (D&C). But now, as hysteroscopy skills improve, diagnosis, and where appropriate treatment, can be undertaken via hysteroscopy alone.

Orthopaedic conditions. Use of scopes in orthopaedics has been almost exclusively to observe the inside of joints. In the past this necessitated an open procedure and all the complications that often arose. Within the knee, conditions that may be treated via an arthroscope include:

- damaged cruciate ligament
- torn menisci
- erosion of cartilage
- removal of foreign bodies.

Urological conditions. Urological conditions are not easy to diagnose without a cystoscopy to visualize the bladder; such conditions include:

- recurrent cystitis
- haematuria of unknown origin

- bladder carcinoma
- benign bladder polyps and warts
- bladder stones
- inflammation of the bladder wall.

Visualization allows a correct diagnosis to be made and treatment if required.

Surgical procedures

There is an increasing diversity of MIS procedures being performed within the day surgery department. The most common procedures which take place in day surgery units are briefly described here. Patient dignity and safety in placing in the lithotomy position need to be maintained in the operating room. Under general anaesthetic the patient's arms are tucked at the sides or folded, and legs must be placed into stirrups simultaneously.

Hysteroscopy and related procedures

The uterus can be visualized by entry via the cervix. Therefore dilatation is required, but not as extensively as for D&C for entry of the hysteroscope. To allow visualization, the uterus needs to be distended. This is usually achieved by introduction of either carbon dioxide (CO_2) from an insufflator or sterile fluid such as glycine or Hiskon – a thick viscose medium.

Laparoscopy and related procedures

Visualization of the peritoneal cavity requires space into which to shine light and manipulate structures. This is achieved by creating a pnuemo-peritoneum by filling the peritoneal cavity with a gas to distend the abdominal wall. Carbon dioxide is the normal gas used as it will not support combustion and has the same refractive index as air and hence does not distort the image. This is introduced by a verres needle which is inserted through the peritoneal wall into the cavity prior to insertion of trocars and cannulae. A second port is usually required, to introduce other instrumentation, for example clip applicators for sterilization techniques.

Arthroscopy and related procedures

Arthroscopy and other procedures requiring visualization of joints usually require two small incision points. In the knee, for example, these are usually either side, just below the patella. This allows an entry point for the scope and another for other instruments which can manipulate the internal parts of the joint. Fluid is needed to flush and aid the view; this is introduced via the scope sheath port. Pathophysiology is viewed and if possible treated with instrumentation, for example trimming of ragged / frayed menisci.

Cystoscopy and related procedures

Cystoscopy is one of the most important urological investigative methods, allowing visualization of the bladder, urethra and prostate. The patient

> Patent dignity and safety in placing in the lithotomy position need to be maintained in the operating room. Under general anaesthetic the patient's arms are tucked at the sides or folded, and legs must be placed into stirrups simultaneously.

is put into the lithotomy position before external genitalia are cleansed. The cystoscope is introduced once an obturator and sheath have been inserted to open the urethra. Sterile fluid such as sodium chloride 9% or glycine is introduced to distend and allow visualization of the bladder wall.

Stones 5 mm or less can be removed using a basket introduced into the urethra via the cystoscope cannulae bridge. This entry is also used to perform diathermy of the inner lining of urethra and bladder.

Equipment

Scopes

The average rigid endoscope has a light source ring of fibre optics around glass optics. This is surrounded by a metal tube. At the top there is an optic or video connection. Usually, the scope then needs to go through a sheath, known as a cannula, which is introduced with a trocar. This allows the removal of the scope after entry. On the sheath there are usually ports to allow introduction of gas, fluid and sometimes other instruments.

Endoscopes work by having glass optics at regular intervals down the metal tube, with illumination required at the bottom end to obtain a view. In present designs, glass rods, concave at each end, are sealed into the metal tube with resin.

Trocars and cannulae are either metal or plastic. These allow the entry site to remain open so that a scope can be removed and inserted. Trocars can be blunt or pointed dependent on the entry required.

Verres needles

Verres needles have a blunt spring-loaded obturator that advances as soon as the sharp tip enters the abdominal cavity. This serves to protect the sharp tip from doing damage. The needle is used to introduce CO_2 to the abdominal cavity before insertion of the laparoscopy trocar and cannulae. Disposable versions are now available.

Insufflator

Recommended average insufflation pressure is 15 mmHg; it can range from 8–10 mmHg for a thin female up to 17–18 mmHg for an obese male.

Sophisticated equipment is now available which automatically delivers CO_2 at predetermined flow rates. Such equipment can constantly monitor and display the intra-abdominal pressure. The average insufflation pressure recommended is 15 mmHg, but this can be effectively altered depending on the size of the individual: 8–10 mmHg for a thin female up to 17–18 mmHg for an obese male (Edelman 1993). Alarm features are present to indicate excessive pressure, and a gauge to monitor amount of CO_2 used. An increasing number of machines also have gas recirculation and smoke filtration incorporated to ensure that the laser/diathermy smoke plume does not obscure the surgeon's vision (Hall 1994).

Light source

The light source is usually fitted with a 170–300 W xenon or halogen lamp, designed for use with video equipment and with automatic intensity control. The appropriate fibre optic light cable is essential. Brightness adjustment is also usually present.

Video camera cable and control boxes

The camera cable is required for scopes that have a video connection. It has a camera head (containing a 1-chip or 3-chip camera) on the scope end and a connector on the other for attachment into the control box. Some leads are watertight and so can be immersed in chemical sterilants. Many are not and so require a sterile plastic sheath to cover them before introduction to the sterile field. The camera control box has an automatic system that tries to optimize the exposure at all times, but there is an override if dark areas need to be viewed. The camera control box must be compatible with the TV monitor from which the image will be viewed. There is also a light-control box which controls the light illuminating the surgical area to maintain constant light at all distances (Phillips 1994a).

Care and sterilization

Although rigid endoscopes appear quite sturdy, they are prone to damage from a number of sources. Care must be taken not to place anything on top of fragile instruments or scopes. Often they are packed into sets and, if not protected in boxes, they are prone to being warped or bent through having other sets stacked on top of them. Catching the scope on box lids and autoclave doors causes kinks. Damage can also be caused by faulty cannulae or by the operator pulling the scope around roughly in the cannulae.

> Rigid endoscopes are prone to damage from a number of sources. Care should be taken when autoclaving them. Avoid sudden, extreme changes of temperature.

Factors to look for when checking rigid scopes (Rothrock 1990) are:

- the lens is free from scratches and allows clarity of vision;
- integrity of the sheath;
- mobility of all moving parts;
- the obturator tip protrudes past the end of the sheath;
- integrity of the rubber bungs/tips;
- patency of channels through instruments.

Rigid scopes can also become bent or warped by a sudden change in temperature, e.g. when taking the scope from the autoclave and putting into cold water, or using very hot water to warm up the scope prior to its entering the abdomen. The scope can steam up as a result of being too hot in the autoclave (above 135°C), a particular problem in bench-top sterilizers. Steaming up happens when the resin breaks down and water drives in under pressure, leading to the presence of water between the glass rods. Cidex or similar products can deposit a film on the distal base glass which blurs the view. Glutaraldehyde can crystallize onto the glass if it is not rinsed off thoroughly, because of the heat from the light source.

Before use and between patients, the scope and other instrumentation should be washed in detergent. Wherever possible, instruments must be dismantled to ensure thorough cleaning of inaccessible parts. All of this must be undertaken as per manufacturer's instructions, which may vary slightly from one make to another. Most manufacturers recommend the brushing away of debris with a toothbrush (remember debris may not be visible to the naked eye) from all ports, openings and the bottom lens. Flush all channels with detergent solutions and insert and remove luminal brushes where possible at least three times. If recommended, ultrasonic cleaners should be used (if available) at this point, though one should remember that channels must be filled with fluid. Then rinse and dry thoroughly. Check that each instrument is intact and not missing any washers or screws. Check the integrity of all insulated instruments. Lubricate parts where necessary before sterilization/disinfection. Care must be taken to prevent the use of excessive fluid on electrical products.

> High-intensity light sources may cause visual damage. Always hold the scope downwards when not inserted into the patient. The distal end of the light source or scope becomes hot during use and might cause burns if left on unattended.

Care must be taken with use of the light source. High-intensity light sources may cause visual damage. Therefore always hold the scope downwards when not inserted into the patient. The instrument end of the light source (or the distal tip of the scope if it is attached) increases in temperature during use. This can cause burns on contact with the operator, drapes or patient, so must not be left on unattended. Before turning on or off it is good practice to turn down the light intensity to prevent accidental burns or damage to the eyes of personnel; this can also prevent the bulb from 'blowing' or failing as quickly. Documentation of the halogen or xenon bulb life is also required on some light sources (Phillips 1994a,b).

It is good infection control policy to have, where possible, all equipment autoclaved or ethylene oxide gassed or sterilized with low-temperature steam or formaldehyde. Only heat sensitive items should be treated separately with chemical sterilant (Caddow 1989). Presently there appears to be no acceptable substitute for glutaraldehyde. Its use and safety precautions are discussed, below, in the care and sterilization of flexible scopes.

The CO_2 insufflator also needs care and attention. The attached cylinder must be checked to ensure there is enough CO_2 present for the case and that there is a spare cylinder at hand, (Phillips, 1994a). It is important to ensure that there are filters on the output. These can filter the CO_2 of particles, but, more importantly, prevent blood and fluid tracking back into the machine. The insufflator must be serviced at least once a year to have the regulator valve checked (Greengrass & Cunningham 1995).

The video equipment now present in most operating theatres also needs some skill and understanding to ensure that it is set up and works properly. The television monitors should be set up properly and left with the factory settings. Ideally there must be a good blackout in the theatre to avoid glare on the screen (Phillips 1994b). Ideally all the video equipment, including the light source, should be on one trolley to reduce damage and excessive movement of the equipment. This ensures that only equipment that is compatible is used, and if a lockable cabinet style trolley is used, this increases security of the equipment. Cables must not be twisted or tangled, and care must be given to how staff will circulate around the theatre so that cables leading to sockets are not stepped over.

Advantages and disadvantages of rigid endoscopy

An advantage of endoscopy to theatre staff is that they are less likely to be contaminated with blood. One could also argue that therefore the patient is less likely to be contaminated as there is only a small wound or none at all. For the patient there are the benefits of little or no scarring. For many procedures there is less pain and quicker recovery times because of reduced trauma to surrounding tissues, e.g. muscles of abdomen. Eventually as MIS skills increase, most procedures will take less time and have less morbidity than traditional surgery.

Disadvantages include the loss of the surgeon's sense of touch and feel. The visual field can give the operator problems in judging the depth of field and knowing what is happening outside the field of vision. In patients there is a problem, in abdominal MIS, of shoulder pain due to direct irritation of the diaphragm by the carbon dioxide. Chemical disinfection of camera leads does shorten their life (the plastic O rings disintegrate eventually) and so should really be avoided. Within the theatre environment there is an increased amount of machinery needed with associated leads and wires.

Future trends

This area is developing very fast as a result of technological advances. There are already plans for a 2 mm diameter laparoscope which would allow procedures such as investigation and sterilization techniques to be achieved under local anaesthetic. The technique is still in its infancy, but should lead eventually to a faster turn round of cases and a reduced amount of drugs and recovery for the patient. Although not as yet proven, it is thought that there will be less pain as abdominal muscles will be damaged to a lesser degree. Because the person is awake, it is also thought that less carbon dioxide will be needed.

Other future trends include devices to aid prevention of damage to other organs. As more surgery will be performed on a day surgery basis, devices such as trans-illuminating ureteric stents to prevent damage to ureters during abdominal surgery are being developed (Phipps & Tyrrell 1991). Attempts are being made to redesign camera systems to improve the image and field of vision for the surgeon. This will ameliorate the problems associated with depth of field and extent of vision available.

Training centres are now being developed all over the country to allow surgeons and other theatre personnel to learn the skills required in minimally invasive surgery. This is allowing all staff to develop and become more efficient in using the technology available to the day surgery units. As surgeons themselves become more skilled, leading to less time needed to undertake the procedure and less pain for the patient, there will be more operations which will be considered as day case procedures. Already, some day surgery departments undertake laparoscopic colycystectomy, and laparoscopic hysterectomy may soon be seen as a day case. Future limitations as to what is acceptable as a day case are likely to be governed more by the patients themselves.

FLEXIBLE ENDOSCOPY

Brief overview

Flexible endoscopes have revolutionized the investigation of the whole gastrointestinal tract. They provide relative comfort to the patient which allows these procedures to be performed under local anaesthetic or sedation. It allows the operator a better view as the flexible endoscope can follow the convoluted pathways of internal structures. The inside surface of the GI tract is made of fragile mucosa which are less likely to be damaged or perforated by flexiscopes.

Flexiscopes would not be possible without the development of fibre optics. An optical fibre is a long very fine rod of core glass (thinner than human hair) which is surrounded by a thin coating of a different specification of glass. This arrangement allows rays of light to pass along the rod with negligible light leakage/loss. Glass this fine is very flexible and relatively durable. Fibres grouped together are called a bundle and can be divided into two categories: incoherent and coherent. Incoherent bundles are randomly arranged and banded together at each end. These are usually used to transmit light through cables and in scopes. Coherent bundles have a large number of very fine fibres. Each single fibre is positioned at each end in exactly the same place, thus allowing each individual fibre to carry one component part of the complete image (Greengrass & Cunningham 1995).

Clinical conditions

Clinical conditions appropriate for flexible endoscopy are linked to the tracts from external orifices.

Urological conditions. Urological conditions are not easy to diagnose without a cystoscopy to visualize the bladder. Conditions that often present include:

- recurrent cystitis
- haematuria of unknown origin
- bladder carcinoma
- benign bladder polyps and warts
- bladder stones
- inflammation of the bladder wall.

Visualization allows a correct diagnosis to be made. Urethral stones are often accompanied by severe pain, haematuria, nausea and vomiting.

Gastric conditions. Conditions that require gastroscopy include:

- gastritis or gastric pain of unknown cause
- stomach ulcer
- malaena
- hiatus hernia or symptom such as 'heartburn' and reflux of gastric contents of unknown cause.

These would require gastroscopy to aid diagnosis and ensure correct treatment of the symptoms or pathophysiology. Nutritional support may require the insertion under endoscope of a percutaneous endoscopic gastrostomy tube (PEG).

Bowel conditions.

- changed bowel habit
- blood in faeces

- partial obstruction
- intestinal polyps
- bowel cancer.

Surgical procedure

The nurse/ODP role while the patient is undergoing local anaesthetic or sedation is very important. How the patient is monitored will vary depending on the local policies and practices of the institution. But the principles are similar – monitoring the patient for reactions to drugs and changes in physiological states. Particularly for sedation, baseline vital signs pre-operatively and every 15 minutes during the procedure are required, reporting any changes to the surgeon/operator/scrub nurse. Drugs likely to be used for sedation include diazepam and midazolam. Also, because there is no obvious incision site, documentation of every detail of the procedure is very important.

Because of the manner of anaesthesia, patient psychological support is required throughout the procedure. The individual is very likely to be anxious. It is important to establish a rapport with the patient and encourage her to express concerns and ask questions. Information about what will happen is required, both procedural and sensory (Mitchel 1994). The patient will fear pain but there must be an honest description of what to expect so that the patient will trust the descriptions. A calm, unhurried manner by the nurse/ODP instils confidence in the patient, thus allowing her to verbalize feelings and request repeated explanations if necessary. It is important to remember that the environment is alien to the patient. Support and explanation where necessary should help put her at ease. Personnel must ensure that the requirement for speed to complete the procedure is not at the expense of the psychological needs of the patient.

> The nurse has an important role to play in monitoring the patient for reactions to drugs and changes in physiological states. Patient psychological support is required throughout the procedure.

Playing music (something familiar in an alien environment), taking the patient's mind off the procedure by talking and, if known to the patients, relaxation exercises all help in making the experience a favourable one. This will allow as much cooperation from the patient as possible during the procedure (Rothrock 1990).

Cystoscopy

Local anaesthetic is commonly used in a gel form which is introduced into the urethra first and time allowed for the anaesthetic to take effect, which will vary from patient to patient but will be in the region of 2–5 minutes. The use of warmed solutions for skin cleansing may reduce patient anxiety (Rothrock 1990). The scope is then introduced via the urethra and attached to a light source. To aid vision, sterile water for irrigation is attached and administered by a sterile closed irrigation system. The irrigation bag should be 60–90 cm above the cystoscopy table to maintain correct pressure (Rothrock 1990). Spare bags should always be available, with a close eye kept on the emptying bag. But, for longer procedures, irrigation is often given in tandem. Monitoring return of irrigation, vital signs and pain is required.

The patient having the procedure performed under local anaesthetic is likely to be anxious, partly because she is embarrassed about being handled in a very private place. Also there is the fear of anticipated discomfort of urethral instrumentation, what the diagnosis will be and complications. Therefore explanations must be slow and deliberate (Rothrock 1990), and the nurse/ODP's role is partly to clarify aspects of findings and patient's knowledge. Explanation and ensuring the maintenance of correct positioning during the procedure is also required.

Gastroscopy

Before undertaking the procedure there should be an observation of the quality, depth and rate of respirations, and whether there are problems with airway clearance, swallowing or verbal communication as these may alter during or immediately after the procedure. Teeth, gums and lips should be assessed. Dentures and partial plates should be removed and a rubber mouthpiece may be used to protect teeth.

> The patient is usually positioned on his left side, with a nurse/ODP supporting the head and aiding in the maintenance of the airway. Ensuring the patient remains safely on the trolley or theatre table and does not injure himself is paramount. The patient having this procedure under local anaesthetic or sedation may be particularly anxious since it entails swallowing the scope. How the patient is sedated/anaesthetized should be clearly documented.

The patient is usually positioned on his left side, with a nurse/ODP supporting the head and aiding in the maintenance of the airway. Care with the proximity of the patients eyes must be taken. Obviously if the procedure were under general anaesthetic the anaesthetist would undertake this role. Ensuring the patient remains safely on the trolley/theatre table and does not injure himself during the local/sedated procedure is also paramount. The patient may move, particularly as the scope is passed. Additional padding may be required. How the patient is sedated/anaesthetized must be clearly documented, so that postoperative staff will be aware of potential postoperative swallowing problems.

During the procedure the patient's vital signs must be monitored in adherence with local policy. Often this is done in conjunction with a pulse oximeter, as this will highlight respiratory depression. The nurse/ODP will need to help maintain the airway and the position of the scope in the patient's mouth. As the scope is removed, there needs to be observation for respiratory distress, bleeding and difficulty in swallowing. Assessment and documentation of the gag and swallow reflex must be undertaken (Rothrock, 1990).

The patient having this procedure under local anaesthetic or sedation may be particularly anxious because the procedure involves passing the scope which they will have to swallow. Therefore the nurse/ODP should remain with the patient at all times (usually the individual supporting the head) offering frequent explanations, instructions and reassurance in a calm unhurried manner.

Rectal endoscopy

Before endoscopy is undertaken it must be ensured that a good bowel preparation has been undertaken as per local policy. This is important to obtain good visibility of the inside of the lower GI tract. This is provided by either Picolax or similar products or by some form of enema or suppository. The choice of product will vary depending on the procedure being undertaken.

The patient is usually positioned on her left side with her knees up to her chest. Support in maintaining this position is usually required, particularly if the patient is elderly. A nurse/ODP should be at the scope entry point to assist with lubrication of the scope and rectum and to support the scope once inserted (including preventing the scope retracting once in the rectum). To aid visibility, air will usually be introduced, and water sprayed and suctioned out. As the scope is removed any blood or discharge must be observed and documented.

Often, this procedure is performed under local anaesthetic or sedation as per gastroscopy. If the patient is sedated or under local anaesthetic then support and explanations are important, as explained with cystoscopy and gastroscopy procedures.

Equipment

At the top of a flexible scope there will be an optic or video connection with ports for air/water/instrumentation and light source. There will also be movement knob(s) which control wires that make the distal end move. The fibre bundle which makes up the body of the scope is covered in a durable plastic sheath or coat. There is a coherent fibre bundle for vision surrounded by incoherent fibres to transport light.

Care and sterilization

Instrumentation of this nature requires careful maintenance and cleaning regimes. This is time consuming, but it is crucial that it is done thoroughly. Often, there is a preference to have lists of similar procedures, which necessitates an efficient system of turn round of scopes and associated instruments for the next patient. This can be aided by having at least two scopes so that one can be cleaned, disinfected or sterilized while the other is used on the next patient.

Scopes are fragile though much sturdier than they used to be. Therefore care must be taken when handling them. Awareness of the immediate environment is essential while moving scopes to prevent knocking against surfaces, particularly metal (e.g. troughs, sinks, other instruments). If knocked, this can lead to shock waves through the instrument which can shatter individual glass fibres (which shows as tiny spots when viewed through the scope). Overbending of the scope can also cause fibre breakage and also causes overstretching of the control wires or breaking of the impermeable outer coating.

Careful examination of the scope is necessary at the beginning of each list for obvious malfunctions of scope tip, ports and outer coat. The manufacturer's recommended leak test should also be undertaken at this point, particularly if the scope is to be immersed in any form of liquid. Many manufacturers actually recommend it should be done before each procedure. Attempting to view through the scope is also recommended before the start of the list to observe for any broken fibres which may reduce the quality of the image seen.

Before the first sterilization the scope should be washed, as it is between cases, because during storage bacteria may have collected and grown on

The patient is usually positioned on her left side with her knees up to her chest. Support in maintaining this position is usually required. A nurse/ODP should assist with the lubrication of the scope and rectum and should support the scope once inserted. As the scope is removed any blood or discharge must be observed and documented.

For efficient turnround of patients it is advisable to have two scopes: one is cleaned, disinfected or sterilized while the other is used on the next patient.

Care should be taken not to strike the scope against hard surfaces nor to overbend it. Breakage of glass fibres shows up as tiny spots when viewing through the scope.

Virtually all flexible endoscopes are not heat resistant and therefore have to be chemically sterilized.

or in the scope. Then the preferred disinfection/sterilization regime should be used. Virtually all flexible endoscopes are heat sensitive and therefore have to be chemically sterilized (Greengrass & Cunningham 1995).

Chemical disinfection and sterilization

There are many factors which affect the efficacy of disinfectants (Caddow 1989):

- microbial challenge (numbers and types of organism);
- disinfectant concentration;
- shelf life and use life, i.e. length of active life once opened;
- dilution during use;
- pollution during use with inactivating substances;
- contact with inactivating substances such as
  - organic matter: food, faeces, vomit, etc.
  - soaps, detergents and other disinfectants
  - hard water
  - natural/synthetic materials: cork, rubber, cellulose, various plastics.

Often staff misconceive disinfectants'/chemicals' efficacy and usage. Chemicals in ideal situations are very effective, but, in a theatre/endoscopy environment, these ideal conditions rarely occur. The department disinfectant policy should clearly highlight which disinfectants are to be used and for what purposes, but irrational use of disinfectants is reported to be commonplace (Caddow 1989). Most disinfectants can actually become colonized with bacteria if the disinfectant has been inactivated, used past its shelf life or incorrectly diluted. Staff must be vigilant in their methods and documentation. Dilution/opening dates should be routinely written on bottles to notify the solution's status to all staff. If dates are absent and the solution's history is questionable, the solution must be discarded. Regular updates by a designated member of staff or infection control nurse should occur to emphasize the importance of this policy, as repetition increases compliance (Bowell 1993).

The most commonly used chemical sterilizing agent is glutaraldehyde. For theatre use, a 2% solution is usual; when needed it is activated by a florazine solution. Glutaraldehyde is effective against bacteria, bacterial spores, and viruses.

The most commonly used chemical sterilizing agent is glutaraldehyde. It is supplied commercially as an amber-coloured liquid of acidic pH at various concentrations. For theatre use, a 2% concentration is usually used, which when needed is 'activated' by a florazine solution which turns it alkaline and a distinctive luminous green in colour. In an alkaline state (pH 6–8) and normal room temperature, the glutaraldehyde has present in its solution more free aldehyde groups, which research, described by Block (1991), has shown to be a prerequisite for good biocidal activity. The free aldehyde molecules react with proteins to produce a high biocidal effect (Russell et al 1992). Once alkalinized, glutaraldehyde begins to slowly lose the free aldehyde molecules, so it has a short shelf life once activated. At acid pH glutaraldehyde is a very stable solution which allows it to be stored for lengths of time, although an increase in temperature does produce more free aldehyde in acid solution, thus reducing its shelf life (Block 1991).

Glutaraldehyde can be seen to be an effective disinfectant/sterilizer of heat sensitive equipment with a wide microbial action. It is able to disinfect and sterilize by reacting with protein present in various components of the microbe, although studies have shown that the understanding of this action is not yet complete. Thus, Ayliffe et al (1992) recommend at least 1 hour to compensate for any error, which is supported by the British Thoracic Society (1989).

What is clear is that the glutaraldehyde action is linked to its interaction with protein. All research has shown a powerful binding of the aldehyde to the outer layers of the bacterial cell. It is believed this causes the sealing of the cell envelope, thus killing the bacteria, a fact which is supported by enveloped bacteria's being more susceptible to glutaraldehyde than are non-enveloped. However, the biocidal effect of glutaraldehyde is unlikely to be due to sealing of the cell envelope alone, because of the fast action glutaraldehyde has in killing the cell even in the non-enveloped bacteria. Glutaraldehyde's fast action is due to multiple biocidal mechanisms some of which are still unknown.

The tubercle bacillus is more resistant to chemical disinfectants than are non-sporing bacteria, due to a more resilient outer coating. Because glutaraldehyde is widely used for the cold sterilizing of bronchoscopy equipment that may be contaminated with tuberculosis bacilli, it must have good activity against these (British Thoracic Society, 1989). By the same mechanism as with other bacteria, it is presently believed that exposure to 20 minutes of glutaraldehyde should kill tubercle bacilli. Exposure to glutaraldehyde for at least 1 hour is recommended if atypical mycobacterial infection is suspected (Ayliffe et al 1993)

The ability of glutaraldehyde to kill bacterial spores is, perhaps, its most important property. Spores are considerably more resistant to all forms of sterilization than are the original bacteria, and this is always an important issue when considering the sterilization of theatre instruments (Caddow, 1989). Because of this importance, there is a continuing interest by researchers in this area, as the full extent of glutaraldehyde's action on the spore is not known (Block 1991). Ayliffe et al (1993) note that 2% alkaline glutaraldehyde can kill one million spores of *Bacillus subtilis* in 2–3 hours, although manufacturers are recommending 10 hours for soaking instruments to allow penetration of particularly resistant spores (ASEP 1990, Voigt & Perrin 1993).

Research has confirmed the excellent antiviral activity of glutaraldehyde (Block 1991), which is supported by Ayliffe et al (1993) who report that 2% glutaraldehyde will inactivate viruses, including human immune deficiency virus (HIV), in about 1–2 minutes. Few studies relate to the mechanism of viral inactivation by glutaraldehyde. But, again, one can assume that protein inactivation or change of conformation is an important aspect of its action on viruses (British Medical Association 1989). The only viruses that show resistance and to which glutaraldehyde appears ineffective are prions and 'slow viruses' (Ayliffe et al 1993). As there still is little in the way of documented study of these viruses, this area requires further investigation to acquire more conclusive evidence.

Recommendations There are many recommendations due to the complexity of factors which affect glutaraldehyde's activity. Therefore the author has highlighted important areas for consideration. But although the chemical appears very effective, the process required to use it is complicated. There are a variety of factors that influence the microbial activity of the disinfectant, which if misjudged by users can make the chemical ineffective.

Only use glutaraldehyde for heat sensitive instruments As the solution has many risks and problems, only heat sensitive instruments should be sterilized in the medium, as there are other methods available. Endoscope accessories such as biopsy forceps, cytology and cleaning brushes, dilator, snares and water bottles should be sterilized in the sterilizing and disinfecting unit or bench top sterilizer (Babb 1990), along with respiratory and dental accessories.

Provision of a safe working environment Provision of a safe working environment, particularly with respect to proper ventilation, is a workplace responsibility (Voigt & Perrin 1993). The approach should ensure that effective protocols of working are developed to ensure a balance between effective infection control and the potential exposure of staff and patients to disinfectants and sterilants (Ellis 1990). The health authority is at risk of prosecution by the Health and Safety Executive if it fails to protect staff from exposure to glutaraldehyde (Babb 1990): this is well documented as glutaraldehyde is included in the Control of Substances Hazardous to Health (COSHH) Regulations (1988). Planning of new departments must take these COSHH regulations into account.

Glutaraldehyde is included in the Control of Substances Hazardous to Health Regulations. Suitable gloves and eye protection should be used. Minimize the risk of splashes and of release of fumes into the air; ensure adequate ventilation when pouring and especially if spillages occur. Use containers with tight-fitting lids. Only cold water should be used to flush away spillages.

Protective equipment available to staff To avoid contact with eyes and skin, there should be suitable gloves and eye protection available. Gloves of polyethylene, butyl or nitrile rubber, or surgical latex provide adequate protection. PVC absorbs glutaraldehyde over an extended period and should be avoided. It is recommended that a local exhaust system, goggles and extra long gloves (Marigold 'blue Nitrile' and 'biogel D' – Campbell and Cripps 1991) are used for making up and disposing of glutaraldehyde to prevent respiratory and contact sensitivity (ASEP 1990, Cooke et al 1993).

Glutaraldehyde usage should be well documented As there is no method of checking that the equipment is sterile, it is important to be vigilant in documenting the solution's usage. Bottles or troughs of activated glutaraldehyde should be dated to ensure glutaraldehyde is not being used past its shelf life (Gibbs 1990). Use of the solution should be well documented, which should include how many soaks it has had to perform. Once the solution has performed 100 soaks it should be disposed and new solution made up (Cooke et al 1993).

Contain the glutaraldehyde to reduce risks Glutaraldehyde should not be exposed to heat or ultrasonics as this increases evaporation and produces fumes in the air (Ellis 1990). Ensure containers are secure whilst in transport and keep tight-fitting covers on immersion tanks when not in use. Lids should be replaced on empty glutaraldehyde containers before disposal (Campbell & Cripps 1991). Where possible, all systems should be enclosed to minimize atmospheric contamination. It is surprising how many different types of unsuitable receptacles are used for the soaking of instruments (Leinster et al 1993). Wherever possible automatic cleaning units aids reduction of the risk of skin splashes and contact, and a reduction in vapour concentrations. Gloves should be replaced if broken and rinsed before removal. Staff must endeavour to prevent splashes on forearms (Leinster et al 1993).

Used solution should be diluted on disposal. Drainage systems should be enclosed and preferably directly discharged into the main system without connections from other sanitary points. Most hazards occur when solution is poured, so this should be reduced as much as possible, (Ayliffe et al 1993). Prevention of accidents can be achieved by restricting openings or fitting funnels for pouring. During this procedure adequate ventilation is required (Voigt & Perrin 1993).

Ensure equipment and protocols are present for dealing with spillage Respirators should be available for use when dealing with spillage of 3 litres or more of activated solution, and full protective clothing with long sleeved gloves and goggles should be worn. The area should be ventilated and air extracted if possible. An absorbent product such as Haz-Chem Pig absorbent pillows should be available for large spills and disposed of correctly. Only cold water should be used to flush away spillage and to dispose of the solution (Sedgwick 1994). The Health and Safety executive have advised that the long blue immersion tanks are not suitable, as spillage is much more likely with these (Voigt & Perrin 1993).

Good manual or mechanical disinfection/sterilization systems must be maintained There is a high chance of reinfection with reuse of scopes (Block 1991). It is therefore highly important that good standards in cleaning and sterilization techniques are maintained. More than one scope for an operating list ensures more time for cleaning and soaking between patients.

A good wash in neutral detergent immediately after use removes 99.9% of respiratory pathogens (British Thoracic Society 1989) and the majority of other vegetative bacteria. Therefore thorough cleaning of instruments is important. Staff must adhere to manufacturers' and local infection policy recommendations for cleaning, disinfection and rinsing of instruments (Cooke et al 1993), which should be documented and visible to staff as a reminder. The channels need to be cleaned with a sterilized or disinfected brush (Ayliffe et al 1993).

After cleaning, disinfection and rinsing, endoscopes should be dried (preferably with alcohol) before being stored as per local policy and manufacturer recommendations to ensure no buildup of bacteria while in storage. Troughs and machines must be washed out with each solution change in detergent and hot water to prevent a sticky residue collecting in the corners and edges (Gibbs 1990) which could harbour pathogens.

Staff should be well educated The above recommendations cannot be enforced unless staff are educated regarding the substance risk, precautions and maintenance of good working systems. An appropriate surveillance programme for early detection of the effects of glutaraldehyde should be introduced which should include identifying people exposed to the solution. Education as to the effects of glutaraldehyde, and training in safe disinfection techniques and instruction in the use of safe personal protective equipment/clothing, must take place. Safe working procedures in written form should be given to all staff (Campbell & Cripps 1991).

Advantages and disadvantages of flexible endoscopes

Flexible endoscopes allow many procedures to be performed under local anaesthetic. There is a reduced risk of contamination to patients as usually there is no wound and the scope does not cause so much trauma.

Disadvantages include expense of the instrumentation, particularly for repair once damaged due to the fact that they can be damaged relatively easily and that they require complicated cleaning regimes. More manufacturers are working on autoclavable scopes. Until then the advantages and disadvantages of flexible scopes revolve around their sterilization with gluteraldehyde.

Advantages of glutaraldehyde

Wide microbial activity The main advantage of glutaraldehyde as a form of sterilization is its high microbiocidal activity against bacteria and their spores, mycelial and spore forms of fungi, and various types of viruses including HBV and HIV (Ayliffe et al 1992). It is also effective against mycobacteria though the activity is slower than that for normal bacteria (Russell et al 1992, Ayliffe et al 1993).

Short disinfection time Glutaraldehyde can in 10 to 20 minutes disinfect instruments and scopes, as long as thorough cleaning is performed first (Ayliffe et al 1993). This allows effective disinfection and sterilization without a long wait for an autoclave cycle or time while instruments are taken to the CSSD department.

Ability to sterilize without heat The need exists for a disinfectant or sterilant that does not use heat, since flexible fibre optic endoscopes will not tolerate temperatures in excess of 60°C. Theylene oxide sterilization is too lengthy a process to be used as a between-patient routine (Campbell & Cripps, 1991), so glutaraldehyde is an ideal sterilizing medium for these scopes in that respect.

Non-corrosive to the instruments being sterilized Compared with other chemicals, glutaraldehyde is non-corrosive to metals and other materials such as plastics and rubber. It also lacks deleterious effects on cement and lenses of endoscopes (Block 1991).

Remains active in the presence of organic matter Use of glutaraldehyde for disinfection and sterilization in a theatre environment inevitably means the presence of organic matter such as blood and pus on instruments. Glutaraldehyde appears to have a high resistance to organic matter, which is surprising since it has such a potent action against protein. Block (1991) indicates that the presence of 20% blood serum or 1% whole blood does not appear to adversely effect glutaraldehyde activity.

Good storage life in acid form In acid solution glutaraldehyde can be stored for lengths of time. Therefore the solution need only be activated when required to ensure maximum aldehyde activity (Leinster et al 1993).

Disadvantages of glutaraldehyde

Although the chemical appears to have a number of benefits, its use is fraught with many problems. Chemical disinfection is inherently complicated because of the number and variety of factors that influence the microbial activity of the disinfectant.

Short activated life The solution itself is unstable once alkalinized and has a short activated life of 14 days. This instability leads to eventual polymerization of free aldehyde, resulting in little microbial activity and the possible support of *Pseudomonas* growth (Ayliffe et al 1993). Glutaraldehyde's life can be further reduced by dilution during rinse in machine washers or if more than one hundred scopes have been manually processed through a soak trough (Cooke et al 1993).

Loss of activity in heat The loss of reactive aldehydes in alkaline solution on storage is increased as the solution is heated (Block 1991). This is often never considered in the summer in hot, poorly ventilated endoscopy units.

Has fixative properties Glutaraldehyde's fixative properties are an advantage in some applications of the solution. But, as a sterilizer of theatre equipment, this can be a problem. Any organic matter or other media with protein content present on the surface of the instrument as it is immersed in glutaraldehyde will be bonded to the surface and be very difficult to remove (Cooke et al 1993).

Will only sterilize the surface presented Glutaraldehyde can only treat surfaces that are wetted by the solution. A surface could be protected from glutaraldehyde by a layer of gel or other solution used in the last procedure. With endoscopes, it is sometimes difficult to position them in the glutaraldehyde container so that they remain immersed in the solution and be certain that there are no bubbles in any of the internal channels (Sedgwick 1994).

Equipment needs to be thoroughly cleaned before immersion All materials presented to the glutaraldehyde must be clean, on account of its fixative properties and since only surfaces wetted by glutaraldehyde will be treated. If equipment were covered in gel or organic matter, either the microbial load would be too great for the solution, the microbes would be protected inside organic matter which would now be firmly bonded to the instrument, or the solution would not be able to wet the surface of the instrument due to a layer of gel or other solution used in the last procedure. Cleaning is time consuming, and in the case of flexible scopes, requires some skill. Fibre optic scopes because of their complexity are problematic to clean and one can never be certain that all organic matter and solutions from the last procedure have been removed (Axon et al 1981).

Unable to test the sterility of the instrument There is no indication as to whether the glutaraldehyde has been fully effective (Gibbs 1990). If cleaning has not been effectively done or the solution is old or diluted, this would, over a number of procedures produce an increasing buildup of bacteria as the instrument is incompletely disinfected/sterilized. The microbial load would eventually be too great for the solution to effectively sterilize or disinfect in the normal stated times (Ellis 1992). In other methods there are indicators to suggest the success of the sterilizing technique, such as temperature readings and tape that changes colour.

Misconceptions about glutaraldehyde's ability There is a misconception that glutaraldehyde will sterilize anything, how ever dirty the instrument is, in 10 minutes (Leinster et al 1993). Glutaraldehyde can take anything up to 10 hours to sterilize an instrument (Ayliffe et al 1993). It is therefore surprising that 50% of departments had no justification for using glutaraldehyde, as other quicker and safer processes were available within their department (Campbell & Cripps 1991). This misconception is also evident in the sterilization of rigid laparoscopes which are introduced inside the abdominal cavity and in some departments are only given a 10 minute soak in glutaraldehyde.

Instrument needs rinsing after immersion in glutaraldehyde Poor technique in removing the scope from tanks to sterile water for rinsing can result in recontaminating the scope (Ayliffe et al 1993) without the user's being aware. A sticky residue will be deposited on the scope if it is not rinsed properly. If the instrument is then not dried properly before storage it can harbour bacteria in moist patches on the instrument.

Adversely toxic to staff If the threat to the patient by contamination is not enough, glutaraldehyde is also a threat to the staff who are in regular contact with the solution. Medical staff may be adversely affected by the toxicity of the disinfectant unless it is effectively controlled (Ellis 1990). Direct contact with skin will cause it to stain brown, and on prolonged exposure there is skin irritation and sensitization causing dermatitis. Fumes may cause a stinging sensation in the eyes with excessive lacrymation and nasal irritation. Direct eye contact causes blepharitis, conjunctivitis and corneal injury. Glutaraldehyde's vapour is irritating and may cause respiratory hypersensitivity, particularly on long-term high exposure (ASEP 1990). Other less common reactions include headaches, dizziness and slowed reactions (Gibbs 1990).

Duration of exposure required to trigger a sensitive reaction is not known, and it is likely that it will vary from person to person (Ellis 1990). Once sensitized, staff have to be transferred to work that does not expose them to glutaraldehyde.

Equipment to protect staff is expensive

The cost of installing fume cabinets or exhaust ventilation is very expensive, perhaps prohibitively so (Gibbs 1990), but is strongly recommended as masks give no respiratory protection whatsoever (Ayliffe et al 1992). Scope washer machines are also very expensive to purchase, especially as it is likely that two are needed to cope with the demands of the average endoscopy list of approximately 15 cases (Ayliffe et al 1993).

Risk to patients Glutaraldehyde is too irritant for soaking respiratory equipment (Ayliffe et al 1993), although some areas still do this (Campbell & Cripps 1991, Babb 1990). Care must be taken with asthmatic patients in a theatre room containing glutaraldehyde troughs, as it may cause an attack. Bronchoscopes must be particularly well rinsed to avoid respiratory sensitivity (British Thoracic Society 1989).

Future trends

Looking at the advantages and disadvantages of glutaraldehyde, the future trend should be a search for new chemicals that are less toxic. A number of different products are now available which have claims to be an alternative to glutaraldehyde. Several independent laboratories have been commissioned by the manufacturers to test the efficacy of these new disinfectants, but as yet, user safety and instrument compatibility are not fully known. The two main contenders are peracetic acid (NuCidex, Steris) and chlorine dioxide (Dexit, Tristel), but the professional societies and the Department of Health have not as yet cleared these products as suitable alternatives, because of insufficient time to review all their chemical properties (Babb & Bradley 1995).

As heat is the preferred method of disinfection/sterilization, manufacturers are working on flexiscopes that can reliably withstand heat. Certainly new materials are being developed to make fibres within scopes more robust which, it is hoped, in the long run will be cheaper to produce (Greengrass & Cunningham, 1995).

LASER SURGERY

Brief overview

Lasers have been gradually growing in popularity over the past ten years or so. They are becoming more regularly seen on day surgery units as the laser's applications are becoming better known and surgeons' skills have improved in using this technology. But there are a number of safety aspects and rigorous protocols which must be in place when this technology and related equipment is used.

The word laser is an acronym for: *Light Amplification (by the) Stimulated Emission (of) Radiation.* All types of electromagnetic radiation, including visible, infrared and ultraviolet light, occupy a characteristic range of wavelengths in a spectrum. In the case of visible light, the range of wavelengths corresponds to the spectrum of colours, and the colour of light is determined by its wavelength within that range. In a similar way, if a certain wavelength of light is required to perform a specific surgical task, then an appropriate laser which emits light at that wavelength is selected.

Clinical conditions treatable

Lasers are proving so adaptable that it would be very difficult to list all the different clinical conditions that they can be used to treat. The variety of conditions that are treated with lasers varies from one day surgery department to another, dependent on the availability of equipment and the clinical expertise. For example, they are used to treat dermatological conditions such as port-wine stains and skin lesions, colposcopic conditions such as removal of cervical lesions and in ophthalmic surgery. The laser can even be used via the endoscope for cessation of bleeding and removal of lesions in gynaecological, urological and GI surgery.

Equipment

Laser technology is constantly being developed; new lasers are providing a wider variety of available wavelengths and greater variety in their use. Although there are a variety of wavelengths being used, there are similar components to any laser system (Ball 1990).

Components

Excitation source The excitation source provides energy to the laser head for the production of the laser light. This may be by various means dependent on the type of laser and the way in which it will be delivered. This includes electrical, chemical, flash lamp, radio-frequency or battery energy.

Laser head When the active medium (e.g. argon gas) is energized to produce the photons and laser energy this optical resonator amplifies and directs the laser beam via a system of mirrors at each end of the laser head. This allows the intensity of the laser energy to be propagated. One of the mirrors allows the partial escape of laser energy, which can be focused by a lens or passed into the appropriate delivery system.

Ancillary components These are the additional parts needed to aid laser energy production. They will vary dependent on the laser system. But there will be a console to house the various laser components, a cooling system to prevent the laser from overheating, and in some a vacuum pump to aid delivery of the activating medium.

Control panel This is the source of laser operation which controls, for example, the laser modes, wattages and duration times. Computerization has allowed the panels to become easier to use and more sophisticated of late. The panel should have a 'standby' mode to prevent accidental emission of laser beam when, for example, the foot pedal is activated by mistake. Often there are feedback security systems within the control panel to prevent activation of the laser when all the required components are not correctly in place.

Delivery system This is the device or attachment that transmits the laser energy to the operating site from the laser head. This may be either an articulated arm, or laser fibres, and there may be additional devices to modify how the laser is delivered to the operating site dependent on the type of surgery.

Lasers are identified by their wavelength, and the appropriate wavelength will determine what tissue effects will happen and therefore what type of surgery and delivery system is required. The three most common lasers used today are the carbon dioxide, the Nd: YAG, and the argon laser systems (Ball 1990), which are named after their active medium.

Special instrumentation Special instrumentation that is brushed or coated with a non-reflective finish is required for laser surgery. This prevents unintended damage from reflection of the laser beam by shiny instrumentation. But, only those instruments which will be near the laser impact site need to be specially treated. Instruments with a matt finish are also available to decrease reflectability. Backstops, such as titanium rods, are available to prevent tissue other than that which is targeted from being damaged. Mirrors are also manufactured to direct the laser beam into less accessible areas.

Types of laser

Carbon dioxide lasers The carbon dioxide (CO_2) laser has been the principal laser system available until very recently. It operates in two modes; continuous wave or pulse. The active medium is a mixture of CO_2, nitrogen and helium which is excited by an electrical current to generate the laser energy. This is coupled with a visible helium–neon laser (red) to allow the CO_2 laser beam to be aimed at the target site. The beam is delivered to the target site through an articulated arm with mirrors at its joints. In gynaecological and ENT procedures, the laser energy is delivered to the target area by a micromanipulator which is attached to the operating microscope or colposcope. A small mirror on this manipulator is controlled by a joystick which the surgeon operates to treat the area desired. The laser has the capacity to cut, vaporize and coagulate tissue very precisely. It is absorbed uniformly by light and dark tissue, making results predictable, and it does not scatter easily (Ball 1990). It can be used for free hand surgery with focused hand pieces which are attached to the end of the articulated arm. There is also a CO_2 laparoscope and special beam aligner which can be attached for laparoscopic surgery (Goodman 1994).

Argon lasers The argon laser operates at two wavelengths which are usually transmitted together. It also provides its own green aiming beam, though the latest lasers have helium–neon aiming beams. The energy, produced by excitation of an argon gas, is directed through fixed filters and optical fibres which can be in varying diameters and lengths and are very flexible. Special hand pieces with sculptured tips are available, which enable accurate focusing of the laser energy. This type of laser offers high precision and minimal damage to surrounding tissue and has good coagulation properties. Because of these characteristics, this laser is often used for laparoscopic procedures and opthalmology (Ball 1990, Goodman 1994).

> Argon lasers are often used for laparoscopic and ophthalmological procedures.

Nd:YAG lasers Neodymium: yttrium aluminium garnet (Nd:YAG) is a near-infrared laser available with continuous and pulse modes. As with the CO_2 laser, a helium-neon laser is used as an aiming beam. The laser energy is produced via a yttrium aluminium garnet crystal which is 'doped' with neodymium ions. A xenon flash lamp excites the laced crystal to produce the laser energy. The laser can penetrate tissue up to 6 mm and can coagulate without vaporization if required. It has greater tissue absorption and reaction in darker tissue, so compensation must be made for this whilst operating. These lasers are very portable and can be attached to optical fibres and also to a micromanipulator attached to an operating microscope (Goodman 1994). The laser light can be transmitted through clear fluids or structures (unlike CO_2 laser beams). In urology therefore it is effective through the fluid medium in the bladder. It will pass down rigid and flexible endoscopes, therefore being popular for upper and lower gastro-intestinal endoscopy, pulmonary endoscopy, gynaecological and urological procedures. With fine sculptured fibres it can be used as a cutting instrument which is ideal for precise surgery.

Safety measures and care of equipment

Laser management

If a laser is present and used within the department, then staff should contact and preferably be involved with the hospital laser committee. This group establishes safety standards and ensures that they are maintained during all laser procedures. These should be adopted from the Department of Health's safety standards (1984). It is preferred that at least one laser nurse specialist (LNS) should be nominated from the department to oversee the use of the laser within the department including inspection of any special eyewear. The LNS should attend workshops and report to the laser safety officer (LSO) (Kulkaski 1994). The responsibility of care and management of the laser during the procedure is often assumed by the peri-operative nurse, who therefore must know laser safety procedures, laser beam characteristics, operational aspects of laser mechanics and hospital protocol (Rothrock 1990).

There should be a laser operator who remains with the machine at all times while it is in operation. Therefore it should not be the runner as this is considered unsafe. The laser operator can then if necessary immediately activate the emergency cut-off switch. The operator should be fully trained, conversant with the laser and the unit's laser policies, and be able to enforce them. Laser case documentation is important; a laser log should be completed and detailed information added to patient notes (Ball 1990, Kulkaski 1994).

Staff protection

Eye protection must be worn, as eyes are extremely sensitive to laser radiation. But goggles in themselves can become a hazard if not used correctly, as they give the wearer a false sense of security. Depending on the type of laser, different optical densities are required to protect staff from accidental exposure from a diffuse laser beam. Therefore the eyewear must be labelled with the wavelength (and therefore the laser) against which it will give protection, and its optical density. The eyewear will not protect against direct exposure to the laser beam or diffuse beams from lasers for which it was not designed. Optical protection should be checked, prior to distribution to all staff undertaking the procedure, for scratches, cracking and other damage, and it should be ensured that everyone wears the same optical protection. Lens eye filters are available to go over the optic of

---

Nd: YAG laser light can be transmitted through clear fluids or structures (unlike CO_2 laser beams). In urology it is effective through the fluid medium in the bladder. It will pass down rigid and flexible endoscopes, therefore being popular for upper and lower GI endoscopy, pulmonary endoscopy, gynaecological and urological procedures. With fine sculptured fibres, an Nd: YAG laser can be used as a cutting instrument which is ideal for precise surgery.

The responsibility of the care and management of the laser during the procedure is often assumed by the peri-operative nurse, who therefore must know laser safety procedures, laser beam characteristics, operational aspects of laser mechanics and hospital protocol.

Eye protection must be worn. Different optical densities of eyewear are necessary for different lasers. Eyewear will not protect against a laser beam shone directly into the eye, nor against diffuse light from a laser for which the eyewear was not designed. Goggles are required for a patient who is awake during the procedure, or eye pads placed over the eyes if under general anaesthetic.

an endoscope to protect against laser backscatter for the surgeon. Again this eye filter should be laser specific. Also it should be noted that other members of the laser team will still need to wear eye protection. The patient should not be forgotten; if he is awake during the procedure then goggles are required for him, or protective eye pads should be placed over his eyes if under a general anaesthetic. Although at present it is not always considered necessary in the UK, all personnel should have eye examinations prior to working with lasers to document ocular health. Then, in the event that an individual is exposed or has specific eye complaints, a comparison can be made to ascertain damage.

Smoke evacuation is needed to accompany the procedure to aid visibility, but more importantly to protect the staff from the noxious smoke that is produced when the tissue vaporizes. The smoke evacuation system should be filtered. These filters need to be changed regularly, adhering strictly to manufacturers' instructions. Used filters should be disposed of immediately and with care, as per the hospital's infectious waste policy. High-filtration or laser-resistant masks should be worn during all laser procedures to filter any laser smoke particles not extracted by the smoke evacuation system. They are no longer effective if they become damp and therefore must be changed regularly (Ball 1990, Kulkaski 1994).

> Smoke evacuation is necessary, mainly to protect staff from noxious fumes produced by the vaporization of tissue; the filters in this system need to be changed regularly. In addition, high-filtration or laser-resistant masks should be worn.

Fire safety

Fire safety is very important. The laser must not be used in the presence of combustible materials, such as certain anaesthetics, drying agents and ointments. A jug of sterile saline should be kept on the scrub trolley to extinguish a fire within the boundaries of the sterile field, particularly as there are currently no fire retardant drapes on the UK market. Note that some skin cleansing solutions are made with combustible ingredients. Therefore it is good policy to cleanse then dry the skin prior to activating the laser. Some cleansing solutions that stain the skin may also have some adverse effects on the laser beam because of the interaction of laser and solution dye. Always adhere to manufacturers' guidelines on which solutions can be used. A portable fire extinguisher should be present to put out an electrical fire, and a bucket of water for non-electrical fire. Beware that the patient's hair (including facial hair) can ignite during the procedure, so there should be moist swabs, sponges or towels over areas of hair in close proximity to the target site. Patients should remove all traces of hair spray prior to the procedure (Ball 1990).

> The laser must not be used in the presence of combustible materials. Some cleansing solutions should not be used for laser procedures. Moist swabs, sponges or towels should be placed over the patient's hair close to the target site. Patients should remove all traces of hair spray prior to the procedure.

Control of laser procedure area

The laser procedure area should be controlled. Safety signs should be at all doors leading into the area which should be laser specific. Traffic in and out of the area should be prevented during laser activation and limited during the procedure to those personnel directly involved in the procedure. All windows should be covered with opaque material to block passage of the laser beam. An interlocking door system is advisable, if possible, which will automatically lock the doors while the laser is activated and automatically cut out the laser if doors are opened by force. An audible sound must be heard while the laser is activated (Kulkaski 1994). The foot pedal must only be activated by the surgeon who delivers the laser to the operating site. Only one foot pedal should be available to the surgeon to prevent the diathermy or laser pedal being pressed inappropriately, causing injury or damage (Ball 1990, Rothrock 1990).

Care of equipment

The infrared laser optics on the CO_2 laser tend to be hygroscopic, which means that water vapour can be absorbed into them. Therefore care is needed when cleaning any optics, as otherwise they could be damaged. Pressurized air can be blown onto the lens to remove dust. Soap and water must not be used if the lens is smudged, because this could destroy the lens coating. Personnel must follow manufacturers' guidelines to the letter, which may include the use of a special lens cleaner, absolute alcohol or acetone. Any coated instrumentation used with the laser should be inspected regularly to insure the integrity of the coating. If the coating has been breached then recoating will be required (Ball 1990).

Endoscope precautions

Some precautions are required when using a laser in conjunction with an endoscope. When a fibre is used to deliver the laser, it is important that the fibre extends at least 1 cm from the end of the endoscope. This is to decrease the chance of damage to the end of the scope from laser backscatter. The laser operator must see the laser fibre at a suitable distance from the endoscope end before allowing the laser to be activated. In flexiscopes, the laser fibre must be protected in a sheath because the end of the fibre can damage the inside lumen of the biopsy port as it is passed. The fibre can be exposed past the end of the sheath once it exits at the end of the scope (Ball 1990).

Advantages and disadvantages of lasers

The laser has proved to be a very efficient tool that can cut, vaporize and coagulate tissue with remarkable precision. Lasers are proving particularly advantageous in minimal access surgery, since they are the safest high-power energy sources transmittable through long, deflectable ultra-thin channels, and which can be controllable and tissue selective (Slatkine & Mead 1994). This allows incisions to be made with minimal bleeding, which is particularly useful in endoscopy procedures. Lasers have also allowed treatment of dermatological conditions which were previously difficult to treat.

Presently though, the equipment is still expensive to purchase for a day surgery department which may have other equipment and instrumentation which would be adequate for the surgery. But it has become apparent that a laser is not an essential tool, more a useful addition, as much of this surgery can be performed with uni/bipolar diathermy (electrocautery). It also requires extensive staff training and safety protocols to be set up before the equipment can be used. So, decisions will have to be made by the day surgery unit as to whether the benefits of the laser outweigh the cost and laser management requirements.

Future trends

Laser technology is constantly changing, and new uses are regularly being discovered. This is partly because laser applications are being increasingly adopted as an acceptable form of surgery. For example, the holium: YAG laser is a recently developed laser which is currently opening up new fields in ENT, orthopaedics and urology. The tunable dye laser is also something that could be increasingly appearing on day surgery unit shopping lists. This works by the use of a liquid organic dye which is dissolved in a specific concentration of alcoholic solvent and is exposed to an intense light source (usually an argon laser beam). The dye absorbs the laser light, which can be tuned by insertion of a birefringent crystal to produce the required wavelength of laser. They are already being used in dermatology procedures such as treatment of port-wine stains and for the selective destruction of vascular lesions and malignancies. Although there is presently some limitation as to the spectrum of wavelengths available with the tunable dye laser, technological advances will soon overcome this and will produce one laser that can be used for many more applications than lasers presently available can offer. The expense of laser equipment will eventually be reduced. The development of the diode laser may bring this about, and, as it is significantly less expensive to manufacture, it is believed that they will replace ion lasers by the turn of the next century (Grochmal 1994).

CONCLUSION

Surgical intervention is evolving and developing, giving a variety of operative options to the surgeon, and to the patient. Many of the current innovations have contributed to an increase in the number of procedures that can be undertaken on a day basis.

For nurses caring for patients during the operative phase of the day surgery experience, knowledge of procedure and technology is vital. It is also a very necessary part of the overall knowledge required by the multiskilled practitioner. In making preadmission assessment decisions and providing information, the assessment nurse needs knowledge and understanding of the operative procedure. During the discharge process and in followup care and education, detailed knowledge of the procedure enables the nurse to answer questions with some assurance.

REFERENCES

ASEP 1990 ASEP safety sheet. Galen Ltd
Axon A T R, Banks J, Cockel R, Deverill C E A, Newmann C 1981 Disinfection in upper-digestive-tract endoscopy in Britain. Lancet ii: 1093–1094
Ayliffe G A J, Coats D, Hoffman P N 1993 Chemical disinfection in hospitals. Public Health Laboratory Service, Blackmore Press

Ayliffe G A J, Lowbury E J L, Geddes A M, Williams J D 1992 Control of hospital infection: principles and prevention, 2nd edn. Wright

Ayliffe G A J, Lowbury E J L, Geddes A M, Williams J D 1992 Control of hospital infection: a practical handbook, 3rd edn. Chapman and Hall, London

Babb J R 1990 Chemical disinfection and COSHH. ISSM Journal (Jul/Aug): 9–12

Babb J R, Bradley C R 1995 A review of glutaraldehyde alternatives. British Journal of Theatre Nursing 5(7): 20–24

Ball K A 1990 Lasers: the perioperative challenge. Mosby, St Louis

Block S S (ed.) 1991 Disinfection, sterilisation and preservation, 3rd edn. Lea and Febiger, Philadelphia

Boswell B 1993 Preventing infection and its spread. Surgical Nurse 6(2): 5–12

British Medical Association 1989 Infection Control. Edward Arnold, London

British Thoracic Society 1989 Bronchoscopy and infection control. Lancet ii: 270–271

Caddow P 1989 Applied microbiology. Scutari Press, London

Campbell M, Cripps N F 1991 Environmental control of glutaraldehyde. Health Estate Journal (Nov): 2–6

Control of Substances Hazardous to Health Regulations (1988) Statutory Instrument No. 1657. HMSO, London

Cooke R P, Feneley R C, Ayliffe G A J, Lawrence W T, Emmerson A M, Greengrass S M 1993 Decontamination of urological equipment. British Journal of Urology 71: 5–9

Edelman D S, 1993 Tailor insufflation pressure. Laparoscopy in Focus 2(4): 4

Ellis M J 1990 High level chemical disinfectants. Pharmacy Dialogue (Nov). Barrie Raven Associates

Gibbs J 1990 Glutaraldehyde: handle with care. Nursing Times 86(21): 52–53

Goodman C R 1994 Laser physics. In: Hall F A (ed.) Minimal access surgery for nurses and technicians. Radcliffe Medical Press, Oxford

Greengrass S M, Cunningham M (undated but obtained 1995) Endoscopy. Courtesy of KeyMed (Medical & Industrial Equipment) Ltd, Essex

Grochmal S 1994 The future. In: Hall F A (ed.) Minimal access surgery for nurses and technicians. Radcliffe Medical Press, Oxford

Hall F A (ed.) 1994 Minimal access surgery for nurses and technicians. Radcliffe Medical Press, Oxford

Hirsch N A, Hailey D M 1993 Influences on the introduction and use of minimally invasive therapies in Australia. Australian Clinical Review 13: 89–97

Kulkaski S 1994 Laser safety. In Hall F A (ed.) Minimal access surgery for nurses and technicians. Radcliffe Medical Press, Oxford

Leinster P, Baum J M, Baxter P J 1993 An assessment of exposure to glutaraldehyde in hospitals. British Journal of Industrial Medicine 50: 107–111

Mitchel M 1994 Preoperative and postoperative psychological nursing care. Surgical Nurse 7 (June): 22–25

Phillips K 1994a Minimally invasive surgery. British Journal of Theatre Nurses 4(3): 4–8

Phillips K 1994b Theatre nursing in the video age. British Journal of Theatre Nurses 4(5): 18–19

Phipps J H, Tyrrell N J 1991 Transilluminating ureteric stents for preventing operative ureteric damage. British Journal of Obstetrics and Gynaecology 99: 81

Rothrock J C 1990 Perioperative nursing care planning. Mosby, St Louis

Russell A D, Hugo W B, Ayliffe G A J (eds) 1992 Principles and practice of disinfection and infection control, 2nd edn. Blackwell Scientific, Oxford

Sedgwick J A 1994 Management of glutaraldehyde solutions. South Buckinghamshire NHS Trust, unpublished

Semm K (transl. Friedrich E) 1984 Operative manual for endoscopic abdominal surgery. Mosby, Munich

Slatkine M, Mead D 1994 Lasers. In: Hall F A (ed.) Minimal access surgery for nurses and technicians. Radcliffe Medical Press, Oxford

Voigt N, Perrin S 1993 Cidex: COSHH assessment guidelines. Johnson & Johnson Medical, unpublished

Wickham J 1991 Minimally invasive therapy. Health Trends 23: 6–9

Pharmacological advances

Jill Barker

CHAPTER OVERVIEW

The rapid expansion in day case surgery over the last ten years or so has been made possible by advances, not only in surgical techniques, including minimally invasive surgery, but also in the field of pharmacology. New anaesthetic and analgesic agents have been developed, and these, together with new techniques of administration, have allowed day surgery to progress from short operative procedures on ASA (American Society of Anesthesiology) I and II patients, to longer and more demanding operations, and the ability to treat some ASA III patients this way. This chapter reviews the physiology of pain, the pharmacology and uses of local anaesthetics, and the methods of sedation, including patient-controlled sedation. Discussion of general anaesthesia includes the pharmacology of the drugs used in premedication as well as intraoperatively, describing the different means by which anaesthesia can be maintained. Finally the importance of postoperative pain relief is emphasized together with methods of achieving this.

PHYSIOLOGY OF PAIN

Most pain arises in pain receptors (nociceptors) in the skin and musculo-skeletal system. Pain sensation is then transmitted in the Aδ and C fibres to the spinal cord and on to the brain (see Table 5.1) Aδ fibres carry impulses from superficial nociceptors responding to the pain of pinprick

Table 5.1 Classification of nerve fibres

Nerve fibre	Conduction velocity (m/s)	Neuron diameter (μm)	Characteristics
Aα	60–120	12–22	Skeletal motor, fast sensory from muscle and tendon
Aβ	50–70	4–12	Touch, vibration, light pressure
Aγ	35–70	4–12	Proprioception
Aδ	10–25	4–12	Pinprick, heat >44°C
B	3–30	1.5–4	Autonomic preganglionic
C	<3	<1.5	Tissue damage, pressure, heat

Adapted from Nimmo & Smith (1989).

and sudden heat, and are responsible for rapid pain sensation and reflex withdrawal, while C fibres carry impulses from deeper nociceptors responding to pressure, heat, chemical substances such as histamine and prostaglandins, and tissue damage. They are associated with slow pain sensation and immobilization of the affected part, and the sensation is not easily localized.

The Aδ fibres synapse with cells in laminae I and V of the dorsal root ganglia of the spinal cord. C fibres synapse with cells in laminae II and III, the substantia gelatinosa (see Figure 5.1). Neurones then cross to the opposite side of the spinal cord and ascend in the spinothalamic tract to the thalamus and aqueductal grey matter. Fibres are relayed from the thalamus to the somatosensory cortex of the brain.

The gate control theory of pain was proposed by Melzack and Wall in 1965 to explain how psychological and physiological factors can affect pain transmission. The 'gate' is at spinal level, thought to be in the substantia gelatinosa, and is opened or closed by various neural pathways. The further open the 'gate', the worse the pain (see Figure 5.2). Various nerve fibres contribute to control of the gate:

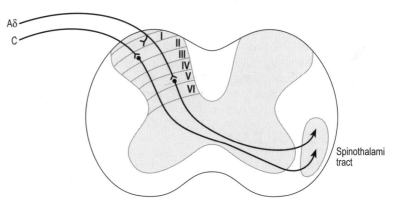

Figure 5.1 Pain pathways in the spinal cord.

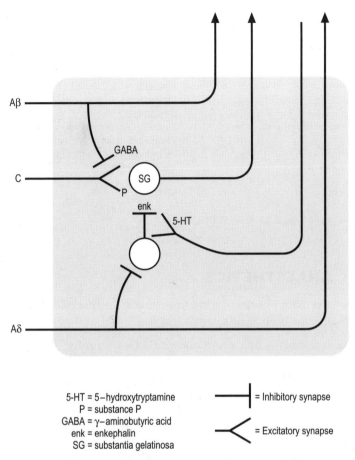

5-HT = 5–hydroxytryptamine
P = substance P
GABA = γ–aminobutyric acid
enk = enkephalin
SG = substantia gelatinosa

———| = Inhibitory synapse

—< = Excitatory synapse

Figure 5.2 Gate control theory of pain. From Yentis et al (1995).

- C fibres from deep receptors, stimulated for example by tissue damage, synapse in the substantia gelatinosa, and open the gate.
- Aβ fibres, which are activated for example by high frequency transcutaneous electrical nerve stimulation (TENS), or by rubbing the affected site, inhibit this synapse presynaptically and close the gate. γ-Aminobutyric acid (GABA) is thought to be the transmitter.
- Aδ fibres subserving temperature, pinprick, acupuncture and low frequency TENS, project cranially via spinothalamic fibres and cause 5HT-mediated descending pathways to close the gate via encephalin-secreting interneurones acting on the target cells. These descending fibres are also affected by mood and emotions, explaining, for example, why an injury during a sports match is not necessarily painful until afterwards.
- Aδ fibres also open the gate by projecting directly onto interneurones to inhibit encephalin secretion.

Pain sensation can thus be modified at many different sites and by ascending and descending pathways as shown in Table 5.2.

Table 5.2 Methods of pain modification

Site of pain stimulus	Method of pain relief
Higher centres	Psychological state
	Placebos
	Opioids
	Dopamine
Dorsal horn of spinal cord	Opioids
	Tricyclic antidepressants
	5-Hydroxytryptamine (5HT)
Aδ & C fibres	Local anaesthetics
Aβ fibres	TENS
Nociceptors	NSAIDs

Adapted from Nimmo & Smith (1989).

LOCAL ANAESTHETICS

There are two main classes of local anaesthetic agents: esters and amides. Examples of ester-type agents are as follows.

- *Procaine* is a short-acting agent and could be useful for day surgery, but is slow in onset and, as with all esters, has problems with systemic toxicity and potential allergic sensitivity.
- *Amethocaine* is mainly used in the UK for topical anaesthesia in the eye. However, a gel formulation has been recently introduced for topical application prior to venepuncture. After a 30 minute application, it has been shown to provide anaesthesia of the skin for several hours (O'Connor & Tomlinson 1995). Amethocaine is too toxic for systemic use.
- *Cocaine* is the only local anaesthetic with vasoconstrictor properties, and as such is a useful topical anaesthetic prior to nasal intubation or operations on the nose.
  The amide local anaesthetic agents are more commonly used. They are less toxic, more stable and have less allergic potential than the esters.
- *Lignocaine* is a particularly versatile drug, being used topically in the form of gels, ointments and sprays, as well as for local infiltration, nerve blocks and spinal and epidural blockade. It has a fast onset and an intermediate duration of action.
- *Bupivacaine* is not suitable for topical application, but otherwise can be used similarly to lignocaine. Although it is slower in onset, it is also longer lasting, and analgesia is obtained with less motor block.
- *Ropivacaine* is a relatively new local anaesthetic agent, similar to bupivacaine but less toxic. It is similar in its onset and in the duration of sensory block, but motor block wears off more quickly (Griffin & Reynolds 1995). It may replace bupivacaine in the future.

Exact speeds of onset and lengths of action are dependent on the site of application and the nature of the block. For instance, the closer the local anaesthetic is applied to the nerves the faster the onset: in the spinal space,

> The amide local anaesthetic agents – e.g. lignocaine, bupivacaine or ropivacaine – are more commonly used. They are less toxic, more stable and have less allergic potential.

Table 5.3 Characteristics and uses of local anaesthetic agents suitable for use in the day surgery unit

Agent	Uses	Onset	Duration	Comments
Cocaine	Topical	Fast	Short	Vasoconstrictor Addictive
Amethocaine	Topical	Slow	Long	High systemic toxicity
Procaine	Infiltration	Slow	Short	Allergic potential
Prilocaine	IVRA	Fast	Moderate	Least systemic toxicity Methaemoglobinaemia in high doses
Lignocaine	Topical Infiltration Nerve blocks Spinal/epidural	Fast	Moderate	Most versatile
Mepivacaine	Infiltration Nerve blocks	Fast	Moderate	Similar to lignocaine Not available in UK
Bupivacaine	Infiltration Nerve blocks Spinal/epidural	Moderate	Long	Sensory-motor dissociation
Ropivacaine	Infiltration Nerve blocks Spinal/epidural	Moderate	Long	Similar to bupivacaine but shorter motor block
Etidocaine	Infiltration Nerve blocks	Fast	Long	Profound motor block Not available in UK

the effect of bupivacaine can be seen in 5 minutes, with the effect lasting 3–4 hours. The larger the volume used for the block, the longer the effect lasts: brachial plexus blocks with bupivacaine take 30 minutes for effect but, because of the larger volumes used, may last for 12 hours. Generally, for postoperative analgesia, a longer-acting agent such as bupivacaine is more beneficial. But if the local anaesthetic needs to have worn off to allow the return of motor function so the patient can return home safely, then a shorter-acting agent such as lignocaine is more suitable. Adrenaline, a powerful vasoconstrictor, can be added to the local anaesthetic to reduce local blood flow and therefore slow the rate of absorption of the agent. This allows a larger dose to be used and prolongs its action. Table 5.3 shows the characteristics of various local anaesthetic agents.

Toxicity

Local anaesthetics are relatively free of side effects if used in appropriate dosage and in appropriate anatomical locations. Toxic reactions can occur from overdosage (Table 5.4 shows the maximum recommended doses) or from accidental intravascular or intrathecal injection.

Signs of toxicity are dizziness, ringing in the ears, tingling in the mouth and blurred vision, progressing to drowsiness, confusion, muscle twitching and convulsions. Loss of consciousness with hypotension and bradycardia and/or respiratory and cardiac arrest can follow. The treatment is supportive with oxygen and diazepam to control convulsions, and endotracheal intubation with ventilation and basic life support when needed.

Table 5.4 Toxic doses of local anaesthetic agents

	Plain (mg/kg)	With adrenaline (mg/kg)
Cocaine	1.5	–
Prilocaine	5–6	8
Lignocaine	3	7
Mepivacaine	5	–
Bupivacaine	2	3
Etidocaine	4	–

Safe administration of local anaesthesia requires resuscitation equipment to be available. The patient should have ECG, blood pressure and pulse oximetry monitoring and should have intravenous access in case of emergency. Aspiration should always be performed prior to injection. It is important to give the local anaesthetic time to work, because if surgery is started before complete analgesia is obtained, it can be very difficult to completely abolish pain sensation.

Use of local anaesthetic agents

Topical application

Topical application of EMLA cream is particularly useful for painless venepuncture in children.

EMLA cream (Eutectic Mixture of Local Anaesthetics) is a mixture of lignocaine 2.5% and prilocaine 2.5% in a 5% oil-in-water emulsion cream. This needs 60 minutes of contact time with the skin for effective analgesia and is particularly useful for painless venepuncture in children. An alternative is amethocaine gel which is effective in only 30 minutes (O'Connor & Tomlinson 1995).

Topical anaesthesia is also useful for eye surgery (amethocaine drops); for analgesia and vasoconstriction in the nose (cocaine paste or solution); prior to endoscopy or intubation (amethocaine or benzocaine lozenges and lignocaine spray); and for urethral catheterization (lignocaine gel).

Local infiltration

Bupivacaine, lignocaine and prilocaine are suitable for infiltration anaesthesia. Operations can be carried out purely under local anaesthesia, or good pain relief can be obtained in many procedures by infiltrating the wound prior to recovery from general anaesthesia (GA).

Intravenous regional anaesthesia (IVRA)

IVRA, or Bier's block, is an effective means of providing analgesia in a limb distal to a tourniquet by injecting the local anaesthetic intravascularly. A cannula is inserted into a vein in the appropriate limb and the limb exsanguinated as far as possible by elevation for a few minutes. A tourniquet is then inflated, and local anaesthetic solution is injected into the cannula. A second intravenous catheter must always be present in an uninvolved arm in case of emergencies. It is more comfortable for the patient if a double tourniquet cuff is used. First the proximal cuff is inflated. Once the block is effective, the distal cuff is inflated over the anaesthetized limb, and the proximal cuff can be deflated. Prilocaine is the local anaesthetic of choice for this block; bupivacaine is cardiotoxic and is not recommended. 40 ml of 0.5% prilocaine without adrenaline is injected into the arm, or 75–100 ml of 0.25% prilocaine for the leg. Analgesia occurs within 10 minutes and lasts as long as the cuff is inflated, and for up to 10 minutes after deflation. It is important that the cuff is not deflated for at least 20 minutes after local anaesthetic injection, to allow the drug to fix in the tissues. Early deflation or inadequate inflation, allowing leakage of the local anaesthetic into the circulation, will lead to signs of toxicity.

Absolute contraindications to IVRA include known allergy to the drug used, sickle cell disease, and infections. Patients should be observed postoperatively for signs of local anaesthetic toxicity, and need a recovery time of at least 2 hours; earlier discharge may lead to vasovagal reactions. Since postoperative pain relief is of short duration, adequate analgesia should be provided prior to discharge.

> In IVRA, analgesia occurs within 10 min and lasts as long as the cuff is inflated, and for up to 10 min after deflation. It is important that the cuff is not deflated for at least 20 min after local anaesthetic injection, to allow the drug to fix in the tissues.

> In IVRA (Bier's block), patients should be observed postoperatively for signs of local anaesthetic toxicity, and need a recovery time of at least 2 h.

Nerve blocks

Various peripheral nerve blocks can be performed specific to the site of surgery, either for surgery solely under local anaesthesia, or as an adjunct to general anaesthesia, providing postoperative pain relief. Examples are ankle blocks, retro- or peribulbar blocks for eye surgery, dental blocks for extractions, penile blocks for circumcisions, and ilioinguinal blocks for hernia repair. Brachial plexus block can be performed for upper limb surgery, and, because of the large volume of local anaesthetic solution needed for this block, can provide analgesia for many hours. The patient needs to be warned to protect the anaesthetized arm until sensation returns.

> Patients having brachial plexus block for upper limb surgery need to be warned to protect the anaesthetized arm until sensation returns.

Central blockade

Spinal and epidural anaesthesia can be used in the day surgery unit.

Spinal anaesthesia involves the local anaesthetic solution's being injected into the subarachnoid space at the lumbar level to provide profound analgesia in the lower part of the body. It is suitable for lower limb and lower abdominal surgery.

In epidural anaesthesia, local anaesthetic is injected outside the dura into the epidural space (see Figure 5.3). The analgesia is slower in onset, but has the advantage over spinal anaesthesia that a catheter can also be inserted into the space to provide continuing analgesia for longer procedures (an attribute of less importance in the day surgery setting). The longer onset time can be a disadvantage in the day surgery unit, slowing patient turnround time, unless a second anaesthetist and anaesthetic room is available for setting up the block while the previous operation is in progress.

Spinal anaesthesia would seem better suited to day surgery practice, but for the potential for postdural puncture headache (PDPH), due to possible leakage of cerebrospinal fluid through the hole made in the dura. The headache may not appear until 24–72 hours after the dural puncture,

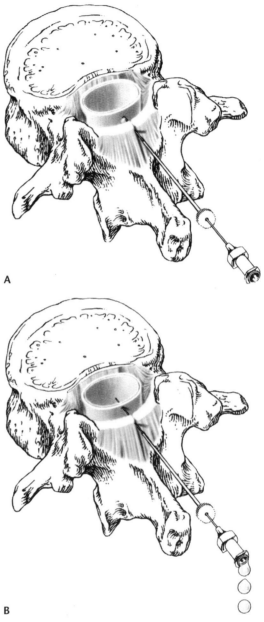

A

B

Figure 5.3 Site of needle placement for (a) epidural and
(b) spinal anaesthesia. Reproduced from Eriksson E 1979
Illustrated handbook of local anaesthesia, 2nd edn.
Lloyd-Luke, London.

Central neural blockade
can be used in day
surgery. Spinal is more
appropriate than
epidural anaesthesia
because of the faster
onset and recovery.
However, there is a risk
of developing PDPH
with a spinal – a severe
headache lasting several
days which is more likely
in young patients,
especially females, who
are mobile
postoperatively.

and many people are reluctant to perform this block in the day surgery
unit, where the patient cannot be observed and the headache treated
appropriately if it should occur. PDPH is a severe headache, worse in the
upright position, which can last several days. It is more likely in young
patients, especially females, who are mobile postoperatively, often the
typical day surgery patient. Studies suggest its incidence is in the order

of 10% (Perz et al 1988), although some give a figure of 37% (Flaatten & Reader 1985). Smaller-gauge needles (25–27 g) with pencil-point tips have reduced the incidence to 2% (Pandit & Pandit 1994), but many people still find this unacceptable and would prefer to use general anaesthesia.

Recovery times from both spinal and epidural anaesthesia are comparable to that for GA, providing short-acting agents such as lignocaine are used for the block. Indeed, some studies have shown that recovery time is actually shorter after regional anaesthesia (Randel et al 1993). There is certainly less nausea, vomiting and drowsiness following spinal or epidural anaesthesia, and immediate postoperative pain relief is better than after GA.

Caudal anaesthesia is epidural anaesthesia given via the sacral hiatus into the caudal part of the epidural space. It is generally used in conjunction with general anaesthesia to provide postoperative analgesia and is especially useful in children having circumcisions or hernia repairs. There is the possibility of leg weakness associated with pain relief, which the children and their parents need to be warned about. This possibility makes it less suitable for adult patients who need to be able to walk out of the unit on discharge.

SEDATION

Sedation provides anxiolysis and some degree of amnesia for the patient undergoing an uncomfortable procedure. Fear is a major stimulus of sympathetic activity, which can lead to hypertension and arrhythmias and can compromise myocardial function. Analgesia is provided, where possible, with local anaesthetic solutions, or, where this is not feasible, for example in colonoscopy, a centrally acting analgesic drug can also be given. At all times, the patient must be rousable and able to respond to commands. Deeper sedation implies anaesthesia, with loss of protective airway reflexes and the need for a practitioner competent in maintaining the airway to be in attendance.

The patient should be monitored with both ECG and pulse oximeter during the procedure, and oxygen should be provided using a face mask or nasal prongs. In all cases where sedation is given, resuscitation equipment should be immediately to hand.

The following groups of drugs can be used for sedation.

1. *Benzodiazepines*, e.g. midazolam, diazepam. These drugs are commonly used for sedation because of their wide margin of safety and ease of administration. Midazolam has no active metabolites and has a shorter half-life of about 1.5–2.5 hours (compared with diazepam's 20–70 hours). With both agents, dose requirements can vary greatly and must be titrated for effect. Smaller doses are required in the elderly (Sanders et al 1989).

   Flumazenil is a specific antagonist to the benzodiazepine group of drugs and can be used to reverse the sedation at the end of the procedure, to allow early ambulation and discharge (Sage et al 1987). Caution must be used, especially after diazepam, as flumazenil is short acting and rebound sedation can occur.

Caudal anaesthesia is useful in children having circumcisions or hernia repairs. Children and their parents need to be warned about the possibility of leg weakness associated with pain relief.

Local anaesthesia should be used wherever possible to supplement general anaesthesia, to provide postoperative pain relief. This can be in the form of local infiltration of the operative site by the surgeon, nerve blockade specific to the site of surgery, such as ilio-inguinal blockade for hernia repairs, or central blockade such as caudal analgesia.

Flumazenil, an antagonist to benzodiazepines, can be used to reverse sedation at the end of a procedure, to allow early ambulation and discharge. Caution must be used, especially after diazepam, as flumazenil is short acting and rebound sedation can occur.

2. *Opioids*, e.g. fentanyl. These can be used on their own for analgesia and sedation, but can cause severe respiratory depression, bradycardia and muscle rigidity. They also cause nausea and vomiting. They are best used in smaller doses in combination with a benzodiazepine to provide some analgesia while allowing the benzodiazepine to provide the sedation.

3. *Anaesthetic agents*, e.g. propofol, methohexitone. Intravenous induction agents can be used in smaller than anaesthetic doses to provide sedation. In practice, propofol is the main agent suited to this type of use, due to its ultra-short action and lack of accumulation. As with all the anaesthetic agents, however, it has a narrow therapeutic window, with the dose needed for sedation being little different from that causing general anaesthesia. Although it can be used effectively and has been used for patient-controlled sedation, it can cause apnoea and cardiorespiratory depression and should only be used by an anaesthetist.

Patient-controlled sedation

Sedative drugs can be administered by bolus or infusion, titrating the effect to achieve the required level of sedation. In practice, however, it can be difficult to judge the exact level required, with the patient either remaining anxious or being given too much and becoming oversedated with consequent longer recovery.

Patient-controlled sedation (PCS) has been recently introduced to overcome these problems, and works on the basis that all patients vary in their requirements, and the patient knows best when he is adequately sedated. If he is still anxious, he can give himself more sedative; if he falls asleep, he stops self-administering the drug. The patient is given a button to press, which causes an infusion pump to inject a set volume of drug into his intravenous cannula. A lockout interval is set, during which time no more drug is given regardless of how many times the button is pressed. This allows for the dose administered to have time for effect. The dose of drug given each time is small, and the lockout time may be only the time taken to inject the dose, often a matter of seconds. Propofol and midazolam have both been used with success (Rudkin et al 1992). An initial bolus dose of sedative is often given by the anaesthetist to achieve the required effect, and the patient then maintains his sedation with top-ups of smaller doses. Alternatively, the patient can self-administer all his sedation, but the small doses available to him with each press of the button mean that the required level of sedation takes longer to achieve.

GENERAL ANAESTHESIA

General anaesthesia (GA) in the day surgery unit must provide rapid onset of adequate anaesthesia for surgery, while allowing fast recovery and return to street fitness, with minimal adverse effects such as nausea and vomiting. There is less leeway in the day surgery setting than with in-patients, where the patient can be allowed to come round slowly and pain, nausea and vomiting can be treated as and when they occur.

Premedication

Premedication is the treatment given prior to an anaesthetic and is generally used for anxiolysis and sedation. Many of the drugs used for this purpose prolong the effect of the anaesthetic and so can delay recovery. Thus, in the day surgery unit, sedative premedication is usually avoided. Indeed, most patients do not need the sedation or anxiolysis provided by the premedication. The combination of a calm atmosphere, full explanations, and short waiting times can go a long way toward reducing anxiety. There are however, short-acting sedative agents which are suitable for use in the day surgery unit.

> In the DSU, sedative premedication is usually avoided. A calm atmosphere, full explanations, and short waiting times can go a long way toward reducing anxiety. However, for the more nervous patient, short-acting sedative agents, e.g. midazolam, can be used.

Sedation

Short-acting sedative drugs have been shown to be compatible with early discharge following day surgery and can be used for the more nervous patient prior to her anaesthetic. Midazolam would appear preferable to temazepam as it has a shorter half-life of 1.75 hours compared with 6 hours; but, in practice, both have been found to be effective with no delay in recovery (Nightingale & Norman 1988).

Oral midazolam 0.5 mg/kg has also been found to be effective in children. It is effective within 30 minutes, and recovery is not delayed (Feld et al 1990). However, as with adults, most children do not need sedation, and are calm at induction given suitable surroundings and the continual presence of their parents.

Anxiolysis

Reduction in anxiety levels without associated sedation can sometimes be obtained with beta-blockers. Various agents have been evaluated. One study (Dyck & Chung 1991) showed no difference in anxiolysis with propranolol, diazepam or placebo; another (MacKenzie 1991) showed good effect with the short-acting beta-blocker timolol.

Analgesia

Non-steroidal anti-inflammatory drugs (NSAIDs) are effective analgesic agents often used in day surgery in preference to opioids, as they avoid the side effects of nausea, vomiting and respiratory depression. They act by inhibiting the enzyme cyclo-oxygenase and thus reduce prostaglandin synthesis. Prostaglandins are released from damaged tissue and cause hyperalgesia by sensitizing the nociceptors to pain. Blocking prostaglandin synthesis thus reduces the hyperalgesia, with treatment being more effective if started prior to the tissue damage – in other words, before the start of surgery (Dahl & Kehlet 1991). Thus they are often given as premedication. Aspirin, indomethacin, ibuprofen and naproxen have all been shown to be effective in reducing postoperative pain; three commonly used ones in day surgery are:

> NSAIDs are often given preoperatively to help provide postoperative analgesia. They should not be used in patients with a history of GI ulceration, bleeding disorders, or in those with renal failure. They should be used with caution in asthmatic patients.

- *Diclofenac sodium* – a short-acting NSAID which may be given orally, rectally or intramuscularly (IM); IM injections are painful, and muscle damage has been reported (Power 1992).

- *Ketorolac* – this can be given intramuscularly and also intravenously, so can be used as part of the anaesthetic technique. A dosage reduction has been advised because of reported side effects with ketorolac 30 mg (CSM 1993). The 10 mg recommended dose appears to be efficacious but is shorter acting (Morrow & Milligan 1994).
- *Piroxicam* – this has a half life of over 40 hours and provides prolonged analgesia with a single daily dose. It has a formulation which melts on the tongue and is rapidly absorbed.

NSAIDs should not be used in patients with a history of gastrointestinal ulceration, bleeding disorders, or in those with renal failure. They should be used with caution in asthmatic patients, as a severe attack can be precipitated in some patients.

Antacids

In some patients, it is prudent to administer antacids prior to surgery. Aspiration of stomach contents into the lungs, which can occur during anaesthesia when the protective laryngeal reflexes are absent, can set up a severe inflammatory reaction, which can be fatal. All patients are starved prior to elective anaesthesia in an attempt to prevent this happening, but certain groups of patients are at increased risk. These include the pregnant patient, the obese or those with a hiatus hernia. The antiemetic, metoclopramide, increases gastric emptying; the H_2 receptor antagonist, ranitidine, is used to lower the gastric acidity. Ranitidine is best given twice: once the night before, and again the morning of surgery, but both drugs can be given intravenously or intramuscularly if necessary.

EMLA cream

Applied one hour prior to surgery, EMLA cream can remove the pain of venepuncture, and is particularly useful in children. (See previous section.)

Induction agents

Intravenous agents

Anaesthesia is usually induced intravenously. Propofol is the agent of choice in the day surgery setting.

Anaesthesia is usually induced intravenously. There are several induction agents to choose from, all having the properties of rapid induction of anaesthesia and recovery within a few minutes.

- *Propofol*, a propylphenol presented as a 1% suspension in intralipid, has become the agent of choice in the day surgery unit because of its excellent recovery profile with minimal hangover effects, and low incidence of nausea and vomiting. Induction is smooth, but pain on injection may occur, which can be reduced by the addition of lignocaine. It tends to reduce upper airway reflexes, making early manipulation of the airway, for example insertion of a laryngeal mask, easier than after thiopentone.
- *Thiopentone and methohexitone*, are rapidly acting barbiturate induction agents. Thiopentone is the most commonly used, but it has a long elimination half life and is cumulative after repeat injections.

Methohexitone is more suited to day surgery, but can cause pain on injection and has been associated with involuntary movements and hiccuping as the patient goes to sleep.

- *Etomidate*, an imidazole compound, has a relatively short half life, but is still longer acting than propofol. It is also associated with pain on injection and involuntary movements on induction, and its recovery profile is inferior to those of propofol, thiopentone and methohexitone, with more nausea and vomiting.

Maintenance of anaesthesia Once the patient is asleep, anaesthesia is maintained either by continuing to administer the induction agent as boluses or, more usually, with an infusion, or by inhalation of a volatile anaesthetic agent.

Total intravenous anaesthesia (TIVA) Propofol is the main agent suited to this form of anaesthesia. It is non-cumulative, so that recovery is as rapid and uneventful after an hour or more of infusion as after one induction dose. Recovery from propofol infusion has been compared to that for thiopentone-enflurane anaesthesia, and earlier discharge and less postoperative morbidity has been found (Millan & Jewkes 1988). Propofol may be combined with an opioid such as alfentanil, and the patient is given either oxygen-enriched air or nitrous oxide and oxygen to breathe. The addition of alfentanil and/or nitrous oxide reduces the requirements for propofol, but prolongs recovery and increases the incidence of nausea.

Inhalational agents

Halothane, enflurane and isoflurane are all volatile anaesthetic agents in common use in the DSU. The different physical properties of each agent account for the differences in their potencies, speeds of induction and rates of recovery (see Table 5.5).

The lower the solubility of the agent in blood, shown by the blood:gas coefficient, the more rapid the induction of anaesthesia. Recovery is also likely to be rapid unless the agent is soluble in fat, shown by the oil:gas coefficient, in which case it will be released from the body more slowly.

> Anaesthesia can be maintained with a continuous infusion of propofol or with any of the currently available volatile anaesthetic agents. Isoflurane is the most often used.

Table 5.5 Properties of inhalational agents

	Partition coefficients		MAC[a] (%)	Metabolism (%)	Comments
	blood:gas	oil:gas			
Nitrous oxide	0.46	1.4	104	0	Analgesic but weak anaesthetic agent
Halothane	2.5	225	0.8	20	Hepatotoxicity in repeated anaesthetics
Enflurane	1.9	98	1.7	2	Convulsive properties
Isoflurane	1.4	97	1.2	0.2	
Desflurane	0.42	19	6.0	0.02	Pungent
Sevoflurane	0.6	53	2.0	2	Unstable in soda lime

[a]MAC = minimum alveolar concentration.

The MAC value (minimal alveolar concentration) indicates the potency of the agent and represents the concentration of the agent that prevents movement in response to skin incision in half of the patients studied.

Nitrous oxide. From Table 5.5, it can be seen that the gas nitrous oxide has only weak anaesthetic properties: a MAC value of 104% implies that it is not strong enough to provide anaesthesia on its own. However, it is the only agent which has analgesic properties, and it is a useful adjunct, reducing the concentration of other agents required.

Halothane, enflurane, isoflurane. These volatile agents have minor differences. Isoflurane is the most suited to day surgery, the lower partition coefficients indicating more rapid induction and recovery profiles. In practice, the difference, especially in short operations, is not always obvious clinically; recovery from the cheaper enflurane is also relatively quick. Enflurane has convulsive properties in high dosage and should not be used in epileptics. Halothane has a greater solubility in fat, and, after longer operations, recovery is notably longer. However, it is the least pungent of the volatile agents and so can be used for induction of anaesthesia, for example in children, without inducing coughing. It is metabolized more than the other agents, and its metabolites can cause hepatitis and liver damage, so repeat exposure to halothane within 3 months is contraindicated.

Desflurane. This is a relatively new, volatile anaesthetic agent structurally similar to isoflurane, but with the chlorine atom replaced by fluorine. With low blood and oil:gas partition coefficients, it seems ideally suited to day surgery, as uptake and recovery are extremely rapid; it is also minimally metabolized. It is, however, pungent, and causes coughing and laryngospasm, so cannot be used for induction of anaesthesia. It also requires a special electronic pressurized vaporizer because it has a boiling point close to room temperature (23.5°C) and so cannot be used in standard vaporizers (Wrigley et al 1991).

Sevoflurane. This agent is relatively new to the UK, although it has been in use for some years in Japan. With its blood:gas coefficient of 0.6, induction is rapid, and recovery, while slower than after desflurane, is quicker than with halothane, enflurane or isoflurane. It has a pleasant, non-pungent smell which makes it very suitable for inhalational induction of anaesthesia, usually used in children, but even adults can be induced quickly and easily (Thwaites et al 1997). Its disadvantages lie in the fact that it is unstable in soda lime, and it is metabolized to release free fluoride ions, which have the potential of causing renal damage (Munday et al 1996, Wrigley & Jones 1992).

Muscle relaxants

Muscle relaxation is sometimes required during anaesthesia and surgery in the day surgery unit. This may be to relax the muscles to improve access for the surgeon, or it may be to facilitate endotracheal intubation, required either because access to the airway will be difficult during the operation, as in dental cases; or to control ventilation during laparoscopy or the prone position.

Suxamethonium. This is a short-acting, depolarizing muscle relaxant, extremely useful in the emergency situation because its onset is rapid and intubation is possible within 30 seconds. Its effect wears off in 2–5 minutes. It causes muscle fasciculations prior to paralysis, leading to its major disadvantage of postoperative muscle pains, which occur especially in the neck, back and arms. These can last 3–4 days and are especially common in the ambulatory patient. Suxamethonium is metabolized by plasma cholinesterase, and a small percentage of the population (0.03%) can suffer from prolonged paralysis because of the inheritance of an atypical cholinesterase enzyme.

Atracurium and vecuronium. These are non-depolarizing muscle relaxants, which take 90 seconds to reach good intubating conditions and can be reversed easily after 20–30 minutes. They are competitive neuromuscular blocking agents, competing with acetylcholine (ACh) at the neuromuscular junction. They do not produce fasciculations like suxamethonium and do not have the drawback of muscle pains. Muscle tone would return on its own, given time, but it is usual practice to reverse the relaxation at the end of surgery to speed up recovery and to be assured of full muscle power in the recovery room. Neostigmine, an anticholinesterase, is used to prevent ACh breakdown and provide ACh to compete with the diminishing amount of neuromuscular blocker present. Atropine or glycopyrrinium must be given with the neostigmine to prevent the muscarinic effects of the anticholinesterase, mainly that of bradycardia.

Mivacurium. This is a relatively new muscle relaxant with an onset of action of 90–120 seconds but a short half-life, providing relaxation for 10–15 minutes due to its being metabolized by plasma cholinesterase. It may be useful for short procedures in day surgery, avoiding the myalgia produced by suxamethonium, but patients with an atypical enzyme will show a prolonged block. Its rapid metabolism means that it does not need to be reversed with neostigmine – which can be an advantage, as neostigmine has been shown (King et al 1988) to increase the incidence of nausea and vomiting after surgery.

Rocuronium. This is another newcomer, providing good intubating conditions more rapidly than other non-depolarizing agents. Its length of action is similar to vecuronium.

Opioids

Opioid analgesics are frequently used during anaesthesia. Their use helps provide a smooth induction, reducing the dose requirements of other agents, while providing analgesia during anaesthesia and for a variable time postoperatively. They can, however, increase the incidence of postoperative nausea and vomiting.

Alfentanil. This is widely used in day case anaesthesia because of its rapid onset and short half-life of 1–2 hours. Recovery is thus rapid but analgesia is short lived.

Fentanyl. This is also widely used, with a rapid onset and longer half-life of 3–4 hours, allowing analgesia to last into the immediate recovery period.

Opioid analgesics are frequently used during anaesthesia. They can, however, increase the incidence of postoperative nausea and vomiting and are best used together with an antiemetic. Examples are alfentanil, fentanyl, morphine and pethidine. Tramadol has fewer side-effects.

Remifentanil. This is a new opioid analgesic with an ultra-short duration of action. It is used as an infusion, with no residual opioid activity 5–10 minutes after discontinuing the drug. This means that it helps to provide rapid awakening after surgery, but alternative analgesics need to be given if postoperative pain is anticipated.

Morphine and pethidine. These are still used, but, with slower onset times and longer half-lives, can delay recovery, although having the advantage of providing longer-lasting analgesia.

Tramadol. This analgesic has been relatively recently introduced into the UK, but has been in use in Germany for some years. It is a weak agonist at opioid receptors and acts mainly by promoting the release and inhibiting the reuptake of 5-hydroxytryptamine (5HT). It produces analgesia that is equipotent to pethidine, but without the respiratory depression and dysphoria that pethidine and other opioids produce. Physical and psychological dependence have not been demonstrated but it can cause nausea and vomiting. It comes in both parenteral and tablet form, and may prove to be a useful analgesic for the day-case patient (Anonymous 1994).

ANTIEMETICS

Postoperative nausea and vomiting are unpleasant for the patient and, if protracted, can lead to unplanned admission from the DSU. It should be treated prophylactically in anyone thought likely to suffer – for example, those with previous sickness after a general anaesthetic, or those who suffer from motion sickness. Vomiting is more likely in young, female patients and after gynaecological, abdominal, or squint surgery.

The common reasons for inpatient admission following day surgery are pain, nausea and vomiting. It is very important that these unpleasant side effects are reduced to a minimum. Vomiting is more likely in young female patients, especially if they are anxious, or after gynaecological, abdominal or squint surgery. The incidence is increased after opioid analgesic drugs, and the use of nitrous oxide and neostigmine have been implicated.

Propofol is associated with a low incidence of vomiting and may have an antiemetic effect (Borgeat & Wilder-Smith 1992). Acupuncture at the P6 (pericardium 6) point on the flexor surface of the wrist can also help. The main antiemetic drugs used are metoclopramide, droperidol and ondansetron (Paxton et al 1995).

Metoclopramide. This is a dopamine receptor antagonist acting on the chemoreceptor trigger zone. It also increases lower oesophageal tone and increases gastric emptying. It can cause dystonic reactions, and clinical studies show that it is not universally effective.

Droperidol. This is another dopamine receptor antagonist with strong antiemetic properties, but also the ability to produce dystonic reactions. It is sedative, and recovery times can be significantly prolonged when it is used.

Ondansetron. This is a 5-hydroxytryptamine-3 ($5HT_3$) receptor antagonist introduced for the control of vomiting after chemotherapy and now available for anaesthetic use. Studies have shown it to be highly effective for the prevention of postoperative nausea and vomiting, with no significant side effects (Scuderi et al 1993).

POSTOPERATIVE ANALGESIA

Control of pain postoperatively is important after any surgery, but arguably especially so following day case operations when the patient needs to be comfortable enough to allow him to go home, and, once at home, needs to be able to control his pain with oral analgesics. Combining different methods of analgesia allows the additive effect of the various agents while reducing the side effects. Analgesia needs to be started early, as there is some evidence that pre-emptive analgesia, that is analgesia given prior to the painful stimulus, is more effective than analgesia given later on (Comfort et al 1992).

NSAIDs should be given preoperatively, and provide analgesia without the sedative side effects delaying recovery or the nausea and vomiting associated with opioids.

Local anaesthetic agents should be used wherever possible, either locally into the wound, or more distally as nerve blocks.

Opioid analgesics can be used and, if thought to be needed postoperatively, are best given early, preferably intraoperatively, to allow the patient to wake with minimal pain. The use of long-acting opioids can delay discharge, because of their side effects of sedation, nausea and vomiting; short-acting opioids such as alfentanil may be preferable. If required in the postoperative period, the intravenous route should be used to gain rapid control of the pain. The drug can be given by the physician or by the patient in a patient-controlled analgesia system (PCA). This is similar to patient-controlled sedation (PCS), as discussed earlier, with the patient self-administering small doses of analgesic according to his need. An antiemetic agent can be mixed in the syringe. PCA has been shown to be an effective way of managing patients after surgery, but there are few studies on its use in day surgery patients.

Oral analgesics must be prescribed for the patient to take home, with combinations of drugs being useful for the stronger pain of intermediate surgery. Paracetamol may be sufficient for minor operations, or can be used in combination with codeine (e.g. co-codamol), dihydrocodeine (e.g. codydramol) or dextropropoxyphene (e.g. co-proxamol) for stronger pain relief. The addition of regular treatment for a few days with a NSAID such as diclofenac can provide good pain relief avoiding the side effects of opioids, always remembering that these are contraindicated in asthmatics, renal disorders and those with peptic ulceration (see earlier section). If stronger analgesia is required, oral morphine can be given, or tramadol is as effective with fewer side effects.

Regular analgesia provides much better pain relief than analgesia taken once pain has developed, and it should be encouraged in all patients likely to suffer pain postoperatively.

Of paramount importance is the need to keep in mind that analgesia will be required and that, not only should appropriate techniques be used intraoperatively, but medication must be given to the patient for postoperative use. Full instructions on their use, both verbal and written, must accompany the drugs.

> Combination therapy is the best means of controlling pain postoperatively. Thus drugs with different actions are combined for an additive effect while limiting side-effects. Use NSAIDs preoperatively, opioids during operation, local anaesthetic wherever possible, and regular NSAIDs or tramadol plus codeine/paracetamol combinations for a few days postoperatively.

> Postoperative control of pain is particularly important in day surgery. The patient needs to be comfortable enough to go home and, once there, to control pain with oral analgesics. Analgesia needs to be started early and is best taken regularly for several days. Full instructions, both verbal and written, on the use of the analgesics must be given before discharge.

FURTHER READING

Whitwam J G (ed.) 1994 Day case anaesthesia and sedation. Blackwell Scientific, Oxford

REFERENCES

Anonymous 1994 Tramadol – a new analgesic. Drug & Therapeutics Bulletin 32: 85–86

Borgeat A, Wilder-Smith O N 1992 Subhypnotic doses of propofol possess direct anti-emetic properties. Anaesthesia and Analgesia 74: 539–541

Comfort V, Code W E, Rooney M E, Yip R W 1992 Naproxen premedication reduces postoperative tubal ligation pain. Canadian Journal of Anesthesia 39: 349–352

Committee on Safety of Medicines 1993 Ketorolac: new restrictions on dose and duration of treatment. Current Problems in Pharmacovigilance 19: 5–6

Dahl J B, Kehlet H 1991 Non-steroidal anti-inflammatory drugs; rationale for use in postoperative pain. British Journal of Anaesthesia 66: 703–712

Dyck J B, Chung F 1991 A comparison of propranolol and diazepam for preoperative anxiolysis. Canadian Journal of Anesthesia 38: 704–709

Feld L H, Negus J B, White P F 1990 Oral midazolam preanesthetic medication in pediatric outpatients. Anaesthesiology 73: 831–834

Flaatten H, Reader J 1985 Spinal anaesthesia for outpatient surgery. Anaesthesia 40: 1108–1111

Griffin R P, Reynolds F 1995 Extradural anaesthesia for Caesarian section; a double blind comparison of 0.5% ropivacaine with 0.5% bupivacaine. British Journal of Anaesthesia 74: 512–516

King M J, Milaskiewicz R, Carli F, Deacock A R 1988 Influence of neostigmine on postoperative vomiting. British Journal of Anaesthesia 62: 4031

MacKenzie J W 1991 A novel approach to anxiolytic premedication for daycase patients. Journal of the Royal Society of Medicine 84: 646–649

Melzack R, Wall P D 1965 Pain mechanisms: a new theory. Science 150: 971–978

Millan J M, Jewkes C F 1988 Recovery and morbidity after daycase anaesthesia: a comparison of propofol with thiopentone-enflurane with and without alfentanil. Anaesthesiology 43: 738

Morrow B C, Milligan K R 1994 The use of lower dose ketorolac. Anaesthesia 49: 837

Munday IT, Ward PM, Foden ND, Jones RM, Van Pelt FNAM, Kenna JG. 1996 Sevoflurane degradation by soda lime in a circle breathing system. Anaesthesia 51: 622–626

Nightingale J J, Norman J 1988 A comparison of midazolam and temazepam for premedication of day case patients. Anaesthesia 43: 111–113

Nimmo W S, Smith G (eds) 1989 Anaesthesia, Vol. 1. Blackwell Scientific, Oxford

O'Connor B, Tomlinson A A 1995 Evaluation of the efficacy and safety of amethocaine gel applied topically before venous cannulation in adults. British Journal of Anaesthesia 74: 706–708

Pandit S K, Pandit U A 1994 Regional anaesthesia for outpatient surgery. Ambulatory Surgery 2: 125–135

Paxton L D, McKay A C, Mirakhur R K 1995 Prevention of nausea and vomiting after day case gynaecological laparoscopy: a comparison of ondansetron, droperidol, metoclopramide and placebo. Anaesthesia 50: 403–406

Perz R R, Johnson D I, Shinozaki T 1988 Spinal anaesthesia for outpatient surgery. Anaesthesia and Analgesia 67: S168

Power I 1992 Muscle damage with diclofenac injection. Anaesthesia 47: 451

Randel G I, Kothary S P, Pandit S K, Brousseau M, Levy L 1993 Recovery characteristics of three anaesthetic techniques for outpatient surgery. Ambulatory Surgery 1: 25–30

Rudkin G E, Osborne G A, Finn B P, Jarvis D A, Vickers D 1992 Intra-operative patient-controlled sedation: comparison of patient-controlled propofol with patient-controlled midazolam. Anaesthesia 47: 376–381

Sage D J, Chase A, Boas R A 1987 Reversal of midazolam sedation with Anexate. British Journal of Anaesthesia 59: 459–464

Sanders L D, Davies-Evans J, Rosen M, Robinson J O 1989 Comparison of diazepam with midazolam as intravenous sedation for outpatient gastroscopy. British Journal of Anaesthesia 63: 726–731

Scuderi P, Wechler B, Sung Y-F et al 1993 Treatment of postoperative nausea and vomiting after outpatient surgery with the $5HT_3$ antagonist ondansetron. Anaesthesiology 78: 15–20

Thwaites A, Edmends S, Smith I 1997 Inhalation induction with sevoflurane: a double-blind comparison with propofol. British Journal of Anaesthesia 78: 356–361.

Wrigley S R, Jones R M 1992 Inhalational agents – an update. European Journal of Anaesthesia 9: 185–201

Wrigley S R, Fairfield J E, Jones R M, Black A E 1991 Induction and recovery characteristics of desflurane in day case patients: a comparison with propofol. Anaesthesia 46: 615–622

Yentis S M, Hirsch N P, Smith G B 1995 Anaesthesia A to Z. Butterworth Heinemann, Oxford

Care of children

Anna-Maria Kennedy

INTRODUCTION

Paediatric day case surgery is not a new concept. As far back as the early 1900s Professor James Nicoll pioneered this aspect of surgery. Nicoll set out five key issues on paediatric day surgery:

1. The cost of resources wasted by treatment as an inpatient should be considered; however patients should be selected carefully for day surgery even if controversial.
2. Bedrest for children after day surgery was an impossible and needless achievement, and early discharge prevented cross-infection.
3. Children cared for at home by mothers of average intellect, with domiciliary nursing backup, fared better. To this end, he employed home-nursing sisters to support and advise the mother/family on any potential problems.
4. The possibility of impairment of the child's psychological development as a result of separation from parents should be appreciated.
5. Application of his experiences of early rehabilitation to his adult surgery cases.

These five key issues still hold true and form the basis of paediatric day case surgery today.

The submission of reports and research from various centres of learning and child/family concern groups, led to the formation in 1985 of Caring for Children in Health Services (CCHS) by its parent organizations the Royal College of Nursing (RCN), the British Paediatric Association (BPA), the National Association of Health Authorities and Trusts (NAHAT) and the National Association for the Welfare of Children in Hospital (NAWCH). Research in paediatric day case surgery by the Audit Commission on behalf of the CCHS, resulted in Thornes' *Just for the Day* report (1991). The report sets out 12 Quality Care Standards (see Box 6.1) with 42 principles for all

■ BOX 6.1 A 12–point planned package of care for day case admissions

1. Planned integrated admission to include preadmission, day of admission and postadmission care, incorporating the concept of a planned transfer of care to primary and/or community services.

2. Child and parent offered preparation before and during the day of admission.

3. Specific written information provided to ensure parents understand their responsibilities throughout the episode.

4. Child is admitted to an area designated for day cases and not mixed with acutely ill patients.

5. The child is neither admitted nor treated alongside adults.

6. The child is cared for by identified staff, specifically designated to the day case area.

7. Medical, nursing and all other staff are trained for, and skilled in, work with children/families, in addition to the expertise needed for day case work.

8. Organization and delivery of patient care are planned specifically for day cases, so that every child is likely to be discharged within the day.

9. Building, equipment and furnishings comply with safety standards for children, e.g. safety glass, non-toxic materials.

10. Environment is homely and includes areas for play and other activities designed for children and young people.

11. Essential documentation, including communication with the primary and/or community services, is completed before the child goes home, so that aftercare and followup consultations are not delayed.

12. Once care has been transferred to the home, nursing support is provided, at a doctor's request, by nurses trained in the care of sick children.

paediatric day case admissions, and reinforces the need for careful selection criteria in relation to procedures carried out as day cases. Whenever and wherever a child aged 0–6 years is admitted as a day case, it is suggested that the concept of a planned package of care be adopted. Thorne recommends that such a package should contain the standards listed in Box 6.1, which might also be considered as quality standards.

ENVIRONMENT

Safe, suitable fitments, equipment and toys provide useful stimuli for children who do not need confinement to bed preoperatively. Utilities for parents and a direct dial telephone line are essential.

The environment of the day case unit must be warm and child friendly. Safe, suitable fitments, equipment and toys provide useful stimuli for children who do not need confinement to bed preoperatively. Utilities for parents and a direct dial telephone line are essential. The theatre suite, comprising anaesthetic, theatre and recovery areas, must be child and family oriented.

The staff, headed by a director and administrative manager, must include an appropriate skill mix of nursing staff, experienced in the care of sick children. Play and clerical staff are vital to the smooth running of the unit. Surgeons and anaesthetists must be experienced paediatric practitioners and should not delegate to trainees. A trained, experienced nurse must be available to provide parental support.

PATIENT SELECTION

Elective paediatric day case surgical procedures necessitate strategical preadmission, admission, discharge and followup criteria. Orientation of children and their families in the care environment, with the professionals and staff involved in that care, is essential to the smooth transition from home to hospital to home. This allows for elucidation of problems not manifested in the initial outpatient interview, sometimes rendering a day case procedure unsuitable. Customized and specifically designed paediatric day care units, though desirable, are not the general rule. Nevertheless, units within adult day surgery units must establish separate facilities for paediatric day care procedures.

Current paediatric surgical day care procedures practised vary throughout the country. An overall view of such procedures practised is given in Table 6.1.

Key issues in selection and preparation for children who are to be cared for on a day basis, include:

- suitability of surgery
- physical fitness of the child
- psychological consideration
- psychosocial consideration
- cognitive development of the child
- family commitments.

Preadmission criteria

Preadmission criteria involve appropriate referral by surgeon/physician via outpatient clinic in the first instance. Information is then circulated to staff concerned with the child's admission. A preadmission visit is arranged

Table 6.1 Paediatric surgical procedures performed as day case admissions

General surgery	Herniotomy, hydrocele excision, examination under anaesthesia, rectal biopsy, anal stretch, excision and investigation of lumps and bumps, lymph node biopsy, dermoid cysts, endoscopy, ingrown toenail
Urology	Cystography, circumcision, orchidopexy, division of adhesions, prepucial stretch/plasty, meatal stretch, ureteroscopy, ureterostomy, division of posterior urethral valve
ENT	Division of tongue tied, myringotomy/grommets, examination under anaesthesia, adenoidectomy
Dental	Extractions

1–4 weeks prior to the date of admission, taking into account the age and cognitive development of the child and family commitments. 'The selection of children for day surgery needs to take into account social and psychological factors and this decision needs to be made jointly with the parents' recommends Hogg (1990).

Identifying children as a unique client group is fundamental to child-centred care. Many children attending the unit have neither the emotional maturity nor knowledge or expectation of the treatment they require. Respect for the child's rights and recognition of the child's needs are paramount to a successful outcome.

Physiological parameters

Much controversy surrounds consideration of patient physical status for day case surgery. Preclusion from day case surgery on grounds of age, weight, medical/social/demographic history is largely dependent on the judgement of the experienced anaesthetist, surgeon, general practitioner and hospital senior nursing staff. The American Society of Anesthesiology (ASA) Classification of Physical Status (see Chapter 1) is invaluable in patient selection criteria as the majority of children are ASA Class I or II for day care procedures. The Royal College of Surgeons of England and Wales Guidelines (1992) state that physiological assessment of patients is a more appropriate tool than chronological age assessment.

Age/weight/height

Parents' and children's medical histories are interrelated factors for the experienced anaesthetist in determining suitability for day case surgery. However, exemption of the premature up to 60 weeks of age, who are at risk of developing respiratory problems (apnoea), pervades. Such infants should be designated ASA Class IV according to Steward (1982). Premature infants beyond 60 weeks of age with a medical history of chronic lung disease (bronchopulmonary dysplasia) are excluded from day case surgery. All infants less than 5 kg weight are also excluded, as are growth retard infants, because of the risk of hypothermia and hypoglycaemia associated with their physical status.

PREPARATION

Psychological preparation

In any well-established day case unit, paediatric-trained day surgery nurses are responsible for preadmission visits and play a vital role in assessing the child's interaction/interrelation with the hospital environment. Parents are encouraged to actively participate in their child's care, having first been informed of what to expect before, during and after the operation. A safe, large, play area is made available where the nurse, child, parents/family can discuss in detail all aspects of the operation. Literature, photographs, colourful pictures and toys suitable for different age groups are used to gauge the child's interest. Appropriate literature, easy to read and understand, must be accessible. The nurses and play specialist, by means of direct play, enable the child to gain some control of the situation, while observing the child's reaction and dealing with fears and misconceptions displayed.

Psychosocial preparation

For some parents, day surgery causes additional problems due to family circumstances; for example, no telephone, inadequate housing, over-crowding, long journeys, one-parent family, ethnicity, caring for other dependants, travel difficulties, cost of travel, etc. Therefore, a preadmission visit with referral to the hospital social worker could alleviate the problem. A further referral to the community services, health visitor or social worker may be essential to prevent long-term financial problems. Interpreters and link workers can help to prepare non-English-speaking families to ask questions and express any wishes or anxieties.

Preprocedure considerations

Anaesthetic. Separation from parents should be avoided, as parental presence at induction of anaesthesia is particularly beneficial to preschool children. Very anxious parents, however, may be advised not to accompany their child at this stage, as their anxiety may be transferred to the child, as reported by Bevan et al (1990). The child is allowed a favourite toy for comfort.

> Parents should be present at induction of anaesthetic unless they are very anxious.

Parents should be told that an unexpected intraoperative event such as regurgitation, bronchospasm or hypersensitivity reactions may warrant admission as an inpatient. Moir et al (1987) and Postuma et al (1987) believe that, in centres with well-established day-care programmes, the hospital inpatient admission rate has been only 1–2%. Even so, parents should be made aware of this possibility at the time of admission, to enable them to consider how best to deal with the situation should it arise.

Preoperative fasting. Debate surrounds the length of 'safe' fasting prior to general anaesthesia. Miller (1990) states that prolonged fasting can lead to hypoglycaemia which may present with overt symptoms such as impaired conscious level (commonly drowsiness). If undetected by the primary nurse and other medical personnel, and the patient proceeds to general anaesthesia, it may lead to permanent neurological impairment. This reinforces the need to know your patient and the necessity for nurses to augment preadmission criteria.

As important, is the risk of regurgitation of gastric content and pulmo-nary aspiration under general anaesthetic due to food intake. Farrow-Gillespie et al (1988) advocated relatively large volumes of fluid up to 4 hours preoperatively, claiming that fluid, given 2 hours preoperatively, reduced volume of gastric content at time of induction. Splinter et al (1989) demonstrated that fluid given 2 hours before anaesthesia was safe. Clarity on the implications for fasting, verbal and written, should be given to families if postponement or cancellation of operation is to be avoided. There is no nursing supervision at this stage, and information to children and parents, therefore, must be unequivocal.

> Consumption of fluid may be allowed until 4 h preoperatively, fluid may be given until 2 h preoperatively.

Consent. The Children Act of 1989, implemented in England and Wales in October 1991, has profound legislative implications for professional practice. While the act provides for a wider group of people to be potentially able to consent to treatment, the act focuses more on the child's level of understanding and maturity, giving children the power of freedom of choice. Children under 16 years have the right to consent to or refuse medical examination, provided that they have sufficient intellect to understand the implications of treatment. The act provides for a new concept of parental responsibility, including consent to a medical examination. Nurses, health care workers and other professionals need clear guidelines as to who has the onus of parental responsibility, as that person can consent to the treatment and welfare of the child without involving others in the consultation.

Theatre induction. The nurse and play leader escort the children/family around the theatre suite, encouraging children to familiarize themselves with anaesthetic equipment by handling it. A well-equipped play area with music, television, video, toys, games and puzzles helps keep children preoccupied, thus reducing their anxiety. The child/parents/family are encouraged to express any fears or concerns regarding the operation and other aspects of the day of admission. Parents are given an information booklet and children are given their own special booklet, appropriate to age or level of reading. The preadmission nurse will endeavour, as far as feasible, to be the patient's named nurse on admission day – enhancing the practice of the primary nurse concept.

ADMISSION DAY

On admission, a number of personnel meet the child and parents: the primary nurse, play specialist, anaesthetist, members of the surgical team, theatre nurse, ward manager and ward clerks; some will be familiar faces from the preadmission visit. The nurses and play specialists wear 'child friendly' uniforms and, having established a rapport previously, are on first-name terms with the child and family. This lends to a 'consumer friendly' and relaxed environment.

Nurses and play specialists wear 'child friendly' uniforms and are on first-name terms with the child and family.

A preparation programme designed by the team, including nursing and theatre staff, must be adapted to the maturity of the individual child, taking into account the child's previous experiences. Play equipment and facilities should also reflect the needs and interests of children and families from different social backgrounds.

A concise past and present history of the patient's general condition is recorded (and any changes from the preadmission visit noted if applicable). A check should be made that no contact has been made with infectious diseases and that the child is symptom free from chest infection and influenza. Prescribed medication, allergies/peculiarities and other illnesses which may affect postoperative progress are recorded. In the case of allergy, it is prudent to offer the child some form of identification in conjunction with the identity wrist band which every patient wears. Operating gowns are 'child friendly' but, should the child refuse to wear it, the gown is put on in theatre when the child is asleep to counteract child/family stress.

Minimizing distress/trauma to the child/family is a prerequisite for problem-free anaesthesia – leading to speedy and effective postoperative recovery. The anaesthetist, who assesses the child on the ward, ensures that the child/family are informed about the procedure. The surgical team, in addition to this, also obtains informed consent. All professionals involved with children, particularly in the day unit, must understand 'informed consent'.

Anaesthetic/operation/recovery

Anaesthetic practice is based on physical status, ASA I–V (see Chapter 1). The child/parents are welcomed to the anaesthetic room. The child is seated on a parent's lap for a cuddle. The hand chosen for venepuncture, to which EMLA cream has been applied, is discreetly positioned round the parent's waist to back, enabling administration of anaesthesia out of the child's sight. Once asleep, the child is lifted onto the trolley. The anxious parents are ushered away by their supportive nurse to have coffee and then return on the child's awakening.

> The hand chosen for venepuncture, to which EMLA cream has been applied, is discreetly positioned round the parent's waist to back, enabling administration of anaesthesia out of the child's sight.

Recovery. Oxygen is administered until the child awakens. Continuous observations are made. A pulse oximeter is monitored. Fluid is given when the child's condition is satisfactory. The child is transferred to the ward on a trolley, or in a parent's arms if extremely distressed, accompanied by ward and recovery nurses.

Postoperative care. On the ward, child observations are monitored and pain levels assessed by the nurse who administers analgesia as prescribed. The child takes fluid, followed by toast/cereal 30 minutes later.

The child and parents are seen by the surgeon and, circumstances allowing, the nurse will discharge the child 2–3 hours postoperatively. The nurse will give verbal and written discharge advice with followup instructions. If aftercare is required, the nurse will action a referral for paediatric community nursing visits within 24–48 hours.

Discharge

A check list of discharge criteria is as follows.

- Observations remain stable 3 hours postoperatively.
- Child's pain is controlled and child has appropriate analgesia to take home.
- Child is not nauseated or vomiting and has taken food and fluids.
- Child has passed urine postoperatively.
- Assessment of wound site is satisfactory.
- Child is able to walk unassisted.
- Mode of safe transportation has been discussed and accepted by family.
- Clear, concise, verbal and written information pertaining to particular surgery and its aftercare has been accepted and understood by family.

CONCLUSION

Well-established day care units offer high-quality, cost-effective care and are preferred by the majority of families. Children clearly enjoy the care of appropriately trained staff, knowledgeable in the physical and emotional needs of each group. Inherent in this is preadmission, admission, discharge and followup evaluation of standards and stated outcomes within a multidisciplinary framework. This serves to provide a comprehensive tool for audit. Provision of individualized care equivalent to Thornes' 12 Quality Standards (Box 6.1) must be the norm.

Community function

Liaison with community paediatric nurses is essential to high-quality paediatric day care practice. The aims and objectives of the paediatric community nurses are as follows:

- minimize parental/child anxiety
- reduce unnecessary GP and hospital visits
- identify wounds requiring intervention
- encourage family/partnership in care, by teaching and support.

The provision of community paediatric services by healthcare trusts should be mandatory.

FURTHER READING

Action for Sick Children 1987 The emotional needs of children undergoing surgery. NAWCH, London

Campbell I R, Scaife J M, Johnstone J M 1988 Psychological effects of day case surgery compared with inpatient surgery. Archives of Disease in Childhood 63: 415–417

Department of Health 1989 The Children Act. HMSO, London

Morton N S, Raine, P A M 1994 Paediatric day case surgery. Oxford Medical Publications, Oxford University Press, New York

---

REFERENCES

American Society of Anesthesiologists 1995 Classification of physical status. Day care admissions. Vol 7 No 1 Paediatric Nursing pg. 27 Table 4

Bevan J C, Johnston C, Haig M I, Fousignant G, Lucy S, Kirnon B et al 1990 Preoperative parental anxiety predicts behavioural and emotional responses to induction of anaesthesia in children. Canadian Journal of Anaesthesia 37: 177–183

Farrow-Gillespie A, Christensen S, Herman J 1989 Effect of the fasting interval on gastric pH and volume in children. Anaesthesia and Analgesia 67: S59

Hogg C 1990 Setting standards for children undergoing surgery. Action for Sick Children Quality Review Series

Kennedy A M 1995a Preadmission, admission, discharge and community follow-up study at Royal Hospital for Sick Children. Royal Hospital for Sick Children, London

Kennedy A M 1995b Study of a specifically designated paediatric day care unit. Royal Free Hospital, London

Miller D C 1990 Why are children starved? British Journal of Anaesthesia 64: 409–410

Moir C R, Blair G K, Fraser G C et al 1987 The emerging pattern of paediatric day care surgery. Journal of Paediatric Surgery 22: 743–745

Postuma R R, Ferguson C C, Stanwick R S, et al 1987 Paediatric day-care surgery: a 30 year hospital experience. Journal of Paediatric Surgery 22: 304–307

Splinter W M, Stewart J A, Muir J G 1989 The effect of preoperative apple juice on gastric content, thirst and hunger in children. Canadian Journal of Anaesthesia 36: 55–58

Steward D J 1982 Preterm infants are more prone to complications following minor surgery than are term infants. Anaesthesiology 56: 304–306

Thornes R 1991 Just for the day. NAWCH, London

Framework for care in day surgery

Debbie Hodge

CHAPTER OVERVIEW

This chapter aims to provide the reader with an holistic view of the nursing care within the day surgery setting. An overview of the nursing process and frameworks for nursing care are presented, and a specific framework is developed for day surgery nursing practice.

Attention is paid to nursing documentation and the utilization of care delivery systems within a day surgery setting. To enable the reader to assimilate the ideas presented in this chapter into practice, a sample care plan is included.

HOLISTIC NURSING CARE

The nature of nursing, i.e. what nursing is and what nurses do, has been debated with great intensity in recent years, with the result that not one clear definition emerges.

Within the day surgery setting there is a unique opportunity presented to nurses to provide holistic, patient-focused care from preadmission to discharge (and in some instances followup). It can therefore be proposed that the aim of day surgery nursing is to provide the client (patient) and her carers with a nursing service based on her individual needs in an holistic manner from the time of referral to completion of care. To achieve this aim the nurse working in the day surgery unit will require a wide range of knowledge and skills. The areas of knowledge and skill can be considered in line with Carper's (1979) areas of nursing knowledge.

Carper proposed that 'knowing in nursing' comprised four interrelated areas: scientific, aesthetic, personal and ethical (see Figure 7.1). Within this book, empirics and ethical knowledge are dealt with in Chapters 5 and 8. This chapter will focus on the area of knowing in the actual giving of care.

AESTHETIC KNOWLEDGE

The actual giving of care in the day surgery setting is dependent on the nursing skills and knowledge of the nurse. This knowledge will include the utilization of the nursing process in the patient–nurse relationship to affect

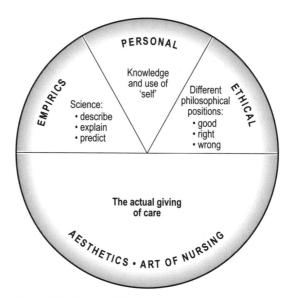

Figure 7.1 Carper's (1979) ways of knowing in nursing.

nursing care outcomes, and a framework (or model) for nursing shaped by the philosophy of care in the day surgery setting. This will guide and inform nursing diagnosis, care, outcome, communication, documentation and influence the nurse–patient relationship. It will also include knowledge of the department's work and systems, along with the technical knowledge related to assessment and procedures undertaken.

The nursing process has been described as a methodical, systematic approach to nursing care which has four stages (Yura & Walsh 1978). The

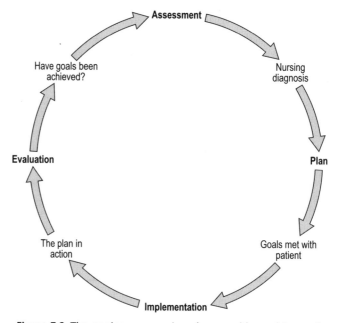

Figure 7.2 The nursing process viewed as a problem-solving cycle.

nursing process is viewed as a problem-solving cycle (see Figure 7.2). Its use in the day surgery setting is expanded in Figure 7.3. The expansion of the nursing process is directly influenced by the progression of nursing care throughout the care episode, beginning with the preadmission assessment and ending with return to the home environment.

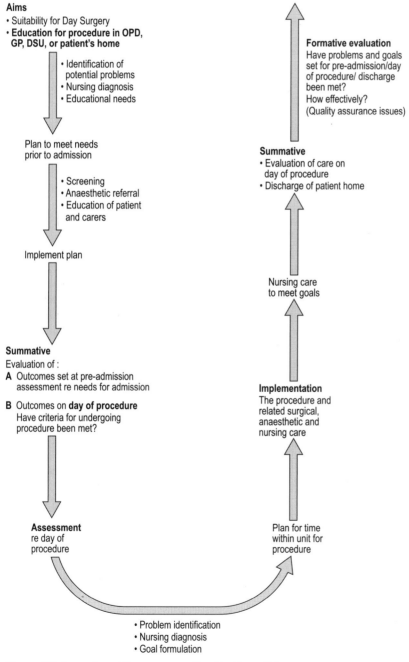

Aims
• Suitability for Day Surgery
• **Education for procedure in OPD,**
  GP, DSU, or patient's home

  • Identification of
    potential problems
  • Nursing diagnosis
  • Educational needs

Plan to meet needs
prior to admission

  • Screening
  • Anaesthetic referral
  • Education of patient
    and carers

Implement plan

Summative
Evaluation of :
A Outcomes set at pre-admission
  assessment re needs for admission

B Outcomes on **day of procedure**
  Have criteria for undergoing
  procedure been met?

Assessment
re day of
procedure

• Problem identification
• Nursing diagnosis
• Goal formulation

Plan for time
within unit for
procedure

Implementation
The procedure and
related surgical,
anaesthetic and
nursing care

Nursing care
to meet goals

Summative
• Evaluation of care on
  day of procedure
• Discharge of patient home

Formative evaluation
Have problems and goals
set for pre-admission/day
of procedure/ discharge
been met?
How effectively?
(Quality assurance issues)

Figure 7.3 Expansion of the process outlined in Figure 7.2.

Preadmission assessment (Chapter 1) focuses on the suitability of the patient for care and intervention on a day basis, the education and preparation of the patient and his escort/carer for both the procedure and aftercare at home. The care process instigated at preadmission assessment is evaluated on two levels and in two distinct areas:

1. the evaluation of the strategies and interventions to assist the patient and her carer/escort to be safely prepared for her procedure, and the suitability of the patient to proceed with care/intervention on a day basis at the time of preadmission assessment;
2. the evaluation at time of arrival for procedure: is the patient properly prepared, does the carer/escort understand his role, have problems (identified at preadmission) been resolved, allowing procedure/intervention to be undertaken.

The second stage of preadmission assessment evaluation criteria forms the assessment phase of the actuality of procedure. This demonstrates the inextricable link between assessment and evaluation, and highlights the similarities in these processes (Figure 7.4).

The key-skills needed in the assessment and evaluation procedure are:

- observation
- communication
- analysis
- critical thinking
- judgement.

Within the process of assessment, these skills are used to determine the suitability of the patient for care/intervention on a day basis and to identify his physical, psychosocial and educational needs in preparation for that care. Data are collected through observation and communication, and comparisons and judgements are made with the admission criteria. Through careful and skilled assessment, the significance of the data presented is

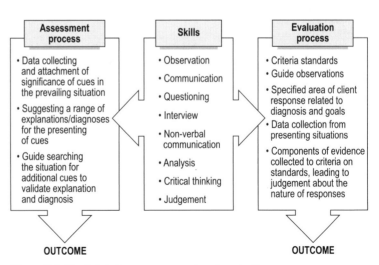

Figure 7.4 The link between assessment and evaluation.

assessed and a range of explanations/diagnoses attempted. The criteria for admission then guide the search for additional data to validate initial explanations/diagnosis. Once validated, the needs of the patient can then be identified and appropriate plans made to ensure safe preparation for the procedure.

The outcome of preadmission assessment is a well-prepared patient (with a confident carer/escort) who, having undertaken preparation at home for the procedure, may undergo that procedure safely.

The evaluation of this initial phase again utilizes the same skills. In this instance, by using criteria standards set for safe preparation for the procedure to be undertaken, as a guide to observation and collection of data from the client's responses, a nursing diagnosis may be reached. Goals may then be formulated from the assessment information in the presenting situation. This evidence is then compared with the criteria, and judgement is made regarding suitability for continuing and the acknowledgement of further needs, both pre- and postprocedure. The outcome from the evaluation of preadmission assessment is the safe preparation of the patient for procedure.

The continuous assessment and evaluation processes within the problem-solving cycle typify the nature of nursing within day surgery care.

MODELS OF NURSING

Care in the day surgery setup involves three phases: preadmission assessment, day of procedure, recovery and followup. To provide continuity of care all nursing staff need a framework or model on which to 'hang' the process of nursing, that reflects their specific values and beliefs and demonstrates patient outcome.

In recent years, there has been much debate regarding nursing models, much of which has been related to the question 'What actually is a nursing model?' Whichever view is taken, i.e. model/theory/framework, all are led in their development and execution by the underlying philosophy of the nurse theorist who formulated the model. In order to understand the viewpoint of the nurse theorist, it is necessary to review the philosophical viewpoints and key tenets of some models/frameworks utilized in nursing practice today.

All frameworks consider the main elements of:

- man, or the individual
- health
- nursing
- environment or society.

What is held true by the theorist for each of these elements is based on his/her philosophy, and the knowledge needed for practice stems from this also.

There have been various attempts to classify the many theories. Riehl-Sisca & Roy's (1980) classification is based on the underlying theory of the model, i.e.

- *development* – based on development theories, e.g. Johnson;

- *system* – based on system theory, e.g. Newman;
- *interaction* – based on interaction theories, e.g. Peplau.

Leddy & Pepper's (1985) classification utilizes four groups relating to the theories that form the model:

- stress and adaptation, e.g. Roy (1984);
- growth and development, e.g. Johnson;
- system, e.g. Newman;
- rhythm, e.g. Fitzpatrick.

Meleise (1985) gave the following classification based on 'Schools of thought':

- needs theories (What do nurses do?), e.g. Orem (1991);
- interaction theories (How do they do it?), e.g. King (1981);
- outcome theories (Why?), e.g. Roy.

By its very nature, no classification of nursing models/theories is definitive, and many overlap. In some instances, a certain theorist's work could be placed in more than one category; this is because, by its nature, nursing revolves around human experiences that are complex and demanding, making demarcation of activity and outcome difficult, thus clouding classification issues.

The question emerges as to which model or framework may be most useful in the day surgery setting. This may be answered by comparing their philosophical viewpoints on day surgery, and the descriptions of the

---

■ BOX 7.1 Orem's self-care model of nursing

- *Background:* This work has been developed through three related theories: namely, self-care deficit, self-care, and nursing systems (Orem 1985). Other nurse theorists influenced her work: Peplau, Orlando and Weidenback, along with Nagels' (1961) work on the structure of science.
- *Man:* a functional, integrated whole with a motivation to achieve self-care. Acts to maintain balance between his/her abilities to achieve self-care and the various demands that are made on his/her self-care abilities.
- *Nursing:* provides a human service, by assisting, helping and intervening; rests with the individual's need for self-care action and the provision and management of it on a continuous basis in order to sustain life and health, recover from disease or injury, and cope with their effects.
- *Health:* state of wholeness or integrity of the individual human being, his parts, his modes of functioning; the capacity to live as a human being within one's physical, biological and social environments and achieve some measure of innate potential.
- *Environment:* a subcomponent of person, and the person and environment are seen as an integrated system related to self-care.

main elements (i.e. man, health, nursing, environment), with those put forward by nurse theorists. A brief overview of the main elements and background notes as put forward by Orem, King, Roper et al, and Roy can be found in Boxes 7.1–4.

For day surgery the four main elements have been described as shown in Box 7.5 (developed with day surgery nurses on ENB N33 course, Barnet, 1994). There are some similarities with the work quoted from established nurse theorists: e.g. interaction (King), biosocial being (Roy), systematic approach to care (Roy), and integrity and return to society (Orem), but no one established framework has the complete answer.

■ **BOX 7.2 King's conceptual framework**

- *Background:* King's work evolved out of a number of theories, notably those of systems theory, perception and interpersonal relationships.
- *Nursing:* a process of interaction between client and nurse where, through perception, goals are set, and, acting on them, transactions occur and goals are achieved.
- *Client:* an individual or group unable to cope with an event or a health problem while interacting with the environment.
- *Health:* the ability to perform the activities of daily living in one's usual roles, a dynamic life experience of continuous adjustment to environmental stressors through optimum use of resources.
- *Environment:* any social system in society, in which there are dynamic forces that influence behaviour, interaction, perception and health.

■ **BOX 7.3 Roper et al's model for nursing**

- *Man:* the client as an individual engages in 12 Activities of Living (ALs) throughout the life span and moves from a state of dependence to independence according to age, circumstances and environment. Man is finite.
- *Nursing:* concerned with helping people to prevent, alleviate, solve or cope with problems related to their ALs. Nursing helps a person towards his independent pole of the continuum of each AL, helping him to remain there, cope with any movement towards the dependent, and, as man is finite, helping him to die with dignity.
- *Health:* the ability to carry out the ALs in a manner acceptable to the individual and the society in which s/he lives in order to meet his/her basic human needs.
- *Environment:* viewed in relation to the influence it has on each AL, there being no distinction between internal and external environment. Factors influencing the ALs are physiological, psychological, social, economic and political.

■ **BOX 7.4 Roy's adaptation model of nursing**

- *Background:* this work seeks to extend Helson's (1964) concept of psychological adaptation to nursing. Helson claims that all organisms strive to achieve optimum levels of physiological and behavioural homeostasis, and this view influenced the development of an 'adaptation' model of nursing.
- *Man:* biopsychosocial being in constant interaction with the environment. The recipient of nursing care, a living complex adaptive system with internal processes acting to maintain adaptation in the four aperture modes (physiological, self-concept, role function, interdependency). The person is a whole made up of parts or subparts that function as a unity for some purpose.
- *Nursing:* a science, a developing system of knowledge about persons, that observes, classifies and relates the process by which persons positively affect their health status. A theoretical system of knowledge which prescribes a process of analysis and action related to the care of the ill or potentially ill person. A practice discipline using a nursing scientific body of knowledge for the purpose of providing an essential service to people, the ability to affect health positively.
- *Health:* a state and process of being and becoming an integrated and whole person. Lack of integration represents lack of health.
- *Environment:* all conditions, circumstances and influences surrounding and affecting the development and behaviour of individuals or groups; input into the person as an adaptive system involving both internal and external factors, categorized as focal, contextual and residual stimuli.

■ **BOX 7.5 Elements of a nursing framework for day surgery**

- *Man:* a unique biosocial complex human being who has individual needs of a spiritual, physical, social and psychological nature, which when addressed will:
  1. promote safe preparation for surgery and care in the unit and
  2. promote re-integration to role and society following discharge from the unit.
- *Nursing:* achieved through partnership and interaction using a systematic approach to care to promote a safe and speedy return to role and society by the patient; the nurse is a specialist in the area of day surgery and an expert communicator and educator.
- *Environment:* provides a feeling of safety, reassurance, comfort and expertise.
- *Health:* the integration and re-integration following surgery to the individual's usual role and society.

In the day surgery setting, there is then an amalgamation of different perspectives, and these culminate in

an interactive framework that promotes partnership in care, utilizing support and education, with technical nursing skills in a reassuring and safe environment, the aim of which is to provide the patient (and his/her carer) with knowledge and skill to be prepared for the procedure required and continued care at home.

This is demonstrated in Table 7.1, which sets out the underpinning ideals that follow patient progression, – from establishing a partnership in care, to the ending of that relationship. The assimilation of these ideas into a practice content can raise many problems, as witnessed by the use of more established frameworks in a variety of practice settings.

SAMPLE CARE PLAN

The usefulness of any framework is dependent on its capacity for practical implementation. The Hodge framework is utilized through the following care plan which puts into practice the ideas embedded in the framework. For this exercise a 'patient profile' is used (see Box 7.6), and care documentation is developed. Figure 7.5 (pp 152–156) shows an outline of Andrew's care cycle, linking care phases, values and beliefs along with the documentation process.

The documentation process is expanded in a sample 'care plan', based on Andrew's care and linked with the key aspects of care documentation needed to establish a record of care given. Specific sections within the care plan relate to the criteria for preadmission assessment, operative consent form, intraoperative care phase documentation, and discharge criteria, and are not completed in explicit detail, as the information to be contained within these sections will be very specific to the multidisciplinary team work within a particular unit. The nurse cannot work in isolation, but is a fully integrated member of the multidisciplinary team. In this particular setting the nurse usually takes the lead in organizing and managing the care pathway by integrating specific services and care options to meet patient needs.

The care documentation reflects the multidisciplinary approach in that all care given by all professionals is recorded in one document, enabling ease of communication within the team, ongoing communication of patient needs and outcomes, and a complete picture of care given throughout the patient's stay.

■ BOX 7.6 Patient profile

Andrew Miles, a 47 year old married man with two teenage children has been referred from the outpatient clinic to the day surgery unit for a repair of his right inguinal hernia.

Table 7.1 Hodge framework for care in day surgery (developed 1994)

Care phase	Underpinning Values	Nursing Action	Patient Outcome
Preadmission assessment (suitability of day care surgery)	Man is unique biosocial complex being with individual needs and ability to make own decisions and take responsibility for preparatory and ongoing care	Interaction Partnerships formation Assessment – skills in communication, education, technical assessment	Safe preparation for surgery and in the day surgery unit
Day of procedure (a) Arrival and preparation	Man is unique biosocial being Responsibility for care in preparation	Renewal of partnership through interaction Preparation evaluated	Accurate and safe arrival and preparation
(b) Procedure	Privacy and dignity maintained (psychological and social needs addressed along with acute physical needs related to procedure)	Utilizes technical skills during procedure, continues interaction and communication	Safety and comfort
(c) Recovery	Physical and psychosocial needs met: pain/nausea, fear	Interaction and technical skills	Safety and comfort
(d) Discharge	Physical and psychosocial needs Responsibility for continued care at home Right to remain longer	Educational interaction and communication skills Evaluation of care and patient outcome	Reassurance Integration to home
Follow up (a) Immediate	Awareness of spiritual/ psychological needs Physical disease	Communcative/ interactive Objective assessment/ evaluation of information presented	Reassurance Integration continues
(b) Long-term	End of partnership		Integration to role and society

Each day surgery unit is unique, not only in terms of location and demographic catchment area, but also in terms of patient care groups, utilization patterns and staff and skill mix ratios. Each unit will therefore deliver care in a way that reflects their particular philosophy and meets patient and service needs.

CONCLUSION

Nursing care in the day surgery unit is founded on the patients' need for information and education on which to base safe preparation for care following an operation or procedure as a day case. Key in this process is the patients' responsibility and ability to take the lead in their own care. This chapter has set out to introduce a framework for care that has the patient as the focus of that care and, based on the philosophy of uniqueness and integration, enables both nurses and patients to achieve their own but related outcomes to ensure quality care and health.

Care delivery in day surgery is a complex activity, made more complex by the increasing number and complexity of operations and procedures performed. With this in mind it is critical that an effective communication system is in place that allows all to access information at all times. Through the utilization of a framework based on unit philosophy and the integration of that framework into a multidisciplinary team care document, patients needs and outcomes can be accessed and acted on by all, to the advancement of quality care.

REFERENCES

Carper B A 1979 Fundamental patterns of knowing and nursing. Advances in Nursing Science 1 (1): 13–23

Helson H 1964 Adaptations level theory: an experimental and systemic approach to behaviour. Harper & Row, New York

King I M 1981 A theory for nursing. Wiley, New York

Leddy S, Pepper J 1989 Conceptual bases of professional nursing, 2nd edn. Lippincott, Philadelphia

Meleise A 1985 Theoretical nursing development and progress. Lippincott, Philadelphia

Nagel G 1961 The structure of science. Harcourt Brace and Would, New York

Orem D 1985 Nursing: concepts of practice. McGraw-Hill, New York

Orem D 1991 Nursing: concepts of practice, 4th edn. Mosby, St Louis

Reihl-Sisca J, Roy C (eds) 1980 Conceptual models for nursing practice. Appleton Century Crofts, Norwalk, NJ

Roper N, Logan W W, Tierney A J 1980 The elements of nursing. Churchill Livingstone, Edinburgh

Roy C 1984 Introduction to nursing: an adaptation model. Prentice-Hall, Englewood Cliffs, NJ

Yura H, Walsh M B 1978 The nursing process. Appleton Century Crofts, Norwalk, NJ

BIOGRAPHICAL DETAILS

Name: **Andrew Miles**

Address: **27 Wood Street**

Anytown

Date of Birth:

1st Language: **English**

Next of Kin: **Mrs Jean Miles**

Escort: **Jean**

Care at Home for 24 Hrs: **YES**

Transport: **YES**

Identified procedure to be undertaken: **Repair Hernia**

Weight [**Kg**] Height [**M**]

Meets height/weight criteria **YES**/NO

Interpreter needed: YES/**NO**

Interpreter organised: YES/NO

Action required: **N/A**

Action required: **NONE**

PARTNERSHIP FORMATION

Named nurse: **Debbie Hodge**

Patient's preferred name: **Andy**

INTERACTION/COMMUNICATION

Previous medical history

.

.

.

. as developed by
Multi display team

.

.

.

.

Pre admission assessment
Action required

**NO
ACTION
REQUIRED**

Outcome

Smoking **10** per day

Alcohol intake **5** units per week

Pre admission education

Information given **YES**/NO   Discussed: **YES**/NO

Action needed: **Further copy of procedure information for children**
I accept responsibility for preparation at home for procedure,

I will not eat from **6 a.m.** or drink from **10 a.m.** on the day of procedure

I will operate no machinery or make important decisions for 24 hours.

Signed

Figure 7.5 Suggested format for documentation of care in the DSU (Hodge Framework for Day Surgery Care).

OPERATION CONSENT FORM
As local/unit based information

Consent form completed

Figure 7.5 (contd)

Day of Procedure, re-establish partnership in care.
Escort/Care at home

Patient has organised Escort | **YES**/NO | Action

Care at home | **YES**/NO | Action

Usual pain relief at home | **YES**/NO | | **YES**/NO |

Patient has NOT eaten since | 6 a.m. | or drunk since | 10 a.m. |

Pre-procedure check list   Action required   Outcome

Consent | **YES**/NO |

NBM | **YES**/NO |

Make Up | N/A |

Family | **YES**/NO |

Empty Bladder | **YES**/NO |

Appropriate clothing | **YES**/NO |

Operation site marked | **YES**/NO |

Name Band | **YES**/NO |

(plus other criteria based on local unit practises)

Patient transferred to Operation Room at | 11.30 a.m. | by   Name..

Signature......................................

Patient returned to Recovery at | 12.30 p.m. | by   Name..

Signature......................................

Operation details

Anaesthetic details

Figure 7.5 (contd)

Immediate post-operative instructive

Stage 1 Post-operative care

Outcome   **Action**

Assessment of level of consciousness   Awake and
                                                   Orientated

Maintenance of Air Way   Mainly
                                                   own
                                                   airway

Assessment of Pain   Score (0-5) | 3 | Check analgesic
                                                give as prescribed

          Nausea   Score | 2 | No action needed

Vital signs | P | | BP | | R |

Wound Site | DRY | | OOZING | | LEAKING |

Stage 2 Monitoring of vital signs   See chart - satisfactory and stable

       Pain | Score 2 |
       Nausea | Score 1 |
       Eating and Drinking | Drink given no nausea |
       Elimination | Passed urine |
       Mobilisers | Walked to toilet |
       Wound Site | Remains dry |

Figure 7.5 (contd)

Discharge and follow up

Discharge Criteria   met/not met   action   outcome

-)
-) as directed from   ) all criteria met
-) unit protocols   )
-)   )
-)   )
-)   )
-)   )
-)   )
-)   )
- Information given   YES/NO

- Patient accepts responsibility for care at home **YES - signed Andrew Miles**

- Nurse completing discharge   name ....

                          signature ....

Follow up care

Patient agrees for telephone call on   at home **YES**/NO

                                             action   **phone as per 7 day
                                                       programme**

Patient agrees for telephone call following day   **YES**/NO

                                after three days   **YES**/NO

                                after seven days   **YES**/NO

Action: Follow telephone calls as in 7 day follow up care

Telephone follow up notes: Day 1 pain slight problem (3 on score)
                                      advise re medication

                               Day 3 pain now no problem,
                                      eating drink well and walking
                                      around home and garden

                               Day 7 wound 'itchy' no other problems
                                      although 'tired' advised not to
                                      'over do it'
                                      See G.P. next week

Care cycle completed date name   **D. Hodge**

                          Signature   ....

Figure 7.5 (contd)

Professional considerations

Ian Peate

8

■ CONTENTS

INTRODUCTION

Ethical issues in the day surgery setting are as important as in any other health care setting. Indeed, it could be stated that ethical and professional considerations in day surgery are the basis on which good, effective, quality care is provided. The Code of Professional Conduct (UKCC 1992a) states clearly in its opening paragraph that 'Each Registered Nurse, Midwife and Health Visitor shall act, at all times, in such a manner as to: safeguard ..., serve ..., justify ... and uphold and enhance ...'. If nurses in day surgery settings are to adhere to such principles then they must first recognize the importance of some general concepts which relate to ethical and moral issues. This chapter focuses on five areas which are central to the provision of high-quality care in the day surgery setting:

- accountability
- informed consent
- children's rights
- day surgery nurse as prescriber
- documentation of care.

Accountability, in the context of nursing care, is best described as the nurse (as a professional) being responsible, in both professional and legal terms, for the type and quality of care delivered. Such a concept is regulated in practice in the UK, by the profession, through the auspices of the United Kingdom Central Council which sets the standards for the requirements of the profession: for example, the Council's foremost document The Code of Professional Conduct (1992a). The Code provides a framework to help guide and develop the professional aspect of the nurse's role. It is a statement of generalizations relating to ideals; the nurse, however, is answerable for his/her own actions. The Scope of Professional Practice (UKCC 1992b) was produced in response to the increased demands being made on nurses by nurses to help them extend and expand their role in order to provide safe, effective care. Supplementary documents were formulated in an attempt to help nurses understand and give guidance when specific areas of concern needed clarification, e.g. The Standards for the Administration of Medicines (UKCC 1992c). This document aims to assist practitioners to enhance care and maintain standards of practice. Confidentiality (UKCC 1987) is a supplementary document which is an elaboration of Clause ten of the third edition of the UKCC's Code of Professional Conduct. It aims to aid nurses, midwives and health visitors with individual, professional judgement concerning the complex issues of confidentiality. Finally, the Standards for Records and Record Keeping supplementary document (UKCC 1993) guides practitioners through the difficulties sometimes associated with record keeping and outlines standards expected by members of the professions. There may also be guidelines/protocols or a clinical practice manual specifically produced by day surgery management teams at a local level, the content of which must be known to all practitioners working in the unit. Further regulations are made by practitioners themselves through audit and ongoing measurement of the quality of care provided. Nurses, therefore, in all spheres of practice are answerable, first and foremost, to the patient (and ultimately society) for their actions and omissions. The content of Box 8.1 highlights the issues of professional accountability in the context of the nurse's role.

Professional accountability, therefore, is a complex and potentially problematic area. Nurses often find themselves in a position which brings with it conflict and dilemmas. These dilemmas are often ethical dilemmas. Ethics generally are to do with 'good' and 'right'. In the West there tend to be two dominant schools of belief which govern ethical thinking: deontology and teleology.

ELEMENTARY DISCUSSION ON SCHOOLS OF THOUGHT RELATING TO ETHICAL ISSUES

Deontology is derived from the Greek word meaning duty. It is the actions or deeds of people which are of prime importance here. This perspective suggests that laws and rules dictate how people behave, and their actions should be such that they do not violate the laws and rules laid down. People 'ought' to behave in a manner which ensures that their actions are within the scope of the law. They have a duty. Young (1991) discusses these issues in more detail.

■ BOX 8.1 Elements of professional accountability

Patient/Society

- Ensure patient care is safe and effective
- Provide patient with information that is relevant and *accurate*
- Preserve trust through honest effective communication

Self

- Monitor own practice ensuring that any misconduct (self and/or others) which may harm the patient, is reported and acted upon
- Enhance own practice by keeping abreast of current practice which is research based and up-to-date
- Ensure clinical decision making is based upon sound fact, as opposed to tradition, ritual and hearsay

Employer

- Adhere to the institution's policies and procedures
- Work in a collaborative manner with other members of the health care team
- Adhere to the law of the land with respect to the Health and Safety at Work Act

Profession

- Adhere to the requirements laid down by the profession (The UKCC) in the form of the Code of Professional Conduct
- Behave in such a manner as to uphold the standards laid down by the UKCC
- Report any activities by other members of the profession which may contravene the standards laid down by the UKCC

Teleology, however, is concerned with the outcome of the actions – the consequences. This word is also from the Greek and is concerned with the goals or the end product of the action. Utilitarianism is closely related to teleology. From the Utilitarianist's perspective the main concern is 'the greater good for the greater number', resulting in 'happiness' for all concerned.

These two schools of thought are often used when nurses need to make clinical decisions. They can, however, because of the many different cultures and value systems inherent in a system such as health care, often lead to differences of opinion and disharmony.

In order for nurses to make clinical decisions or to assist them in resolving the ethical dilemmas encountered on a daily basis, they must be familiar with general ethical principles. Thiroux (1980) suggests five ethical principles which nurses need to consider:

- the principle of the value of life

- the principle of goodness or rightness
- the principle of justice or fairness
- the principle of truth telling or honesty
- the principle of individual freedom.

The five ethical principles outlined above will, to some extent, apply and impinge on all ethical/moral dilemmas which day surgery nurses are faced with on a day-to-day basis.

INFORMED CONSENT

Informed consent is the individual's agreement (conditional or unconditional) to a procedure which involves his/her body, mind or spirit, being performed by another(s), that permission being granted in the knowledge that the individual has a realistic understanding of the procedure and its potential outcome.

True informed consent demands that a person shall be given all the relevant information required to make a decision. In the case of day surgery, the person is agreeing to allow something to happen – the operative procedure. Informed consent allows the patient to reach a decision. Prior to this occurring, it must be determined if the person making the decision is capable of such an activity and that s/he understands the information being imparted. If a patient does not give his/her consent for a surgical procedure to take place, the person carrying out this procedure may be found liable in battery. Battery is any intentional touching of another person's body without his/her consent. It is not necessary, in the case of battery, to have to have caused injury to the person in order to be found liable in battery. In some instances, implied consent is permissible. For example, a patient holding his/her arm out when the nurse approaches with the sphygmomanometer is agreeing to the intended forthcoming procedure (implied consent). In the case of surgical intervention in day surgery, explicit consent is vital.

Valid consent

Informed consent can be given either verbally or in a written form. Good practice would dictate that written consent is preferable to verbal consent (Dimond 1995). In order for the consent to be valid, certain factors need to be considered. Tschundin (1992) identifies these as follows.

- Who may give consent?
- What is the competency of the individual consenting?
- Who should provide information to the individual?
- What is the content of the information presented?

Who gives consent?

The legal minimum age for a person to give consent for an operation, in the UK, is 16 years of age. Any individual under that age must have a parent or guardian's consent. This does not negate the nurse's duty to

> Informed consent can be given either verbally or in a written form. Good practice would dictate that written consent is preferable to verbal consent.

> The legal minimum age for a person to give consent for an operation, in the UK, is 16 years. Any individual under that age must have a parent or guardian's consent.

inform and explain to the child (the individual under 16 years of age) about the proposed procedure. The Children Act 1989 requires that regard is given to 'the ascertainable wishes and feelings of the child concerned in consideration of his/her age and understanding'. The minor aged between 16 and 17 years of age, however, requires further examination. Under Section Eight of the Family Law Reform Act 1969, the minor can give valid consent to a surgical procedure. This act states that it is not necessary for a parent or guardian to give consent. It would be wise, however, to gain consent from both minor and parent or legal guardian.

Competency of a patient to consent

In the cases of the elderly, mentally infirm, or the mentally incompetent patient, consent must be given by the patient's relatives or, in some instances, the doctor, who has a duty of care in situations of necessity. However, the doctor (and the nurse) must always act in the best interests of the patient.

The Mental Health Act 1983 makes provision for the patient's doctor to consent to treatment which may include surgical intervention. In such cases, surgical intervention can be performed legally without the patient's consent. However, should such a situation arise, special consent forms are required to be completed in order that treatment of a patient who is unable to consent, because of a mental disorder, is permissible. It must nevertheless be determined that the patient, in the Registered Medical Practitioner's opinion, is unable to give valid consent for an operation. It is considered good practice to discuss any impending surgical intervention with the patient's next of kin (if known). The consent form must be signed by the patient's Registered Medical Practitioner and the Registered Medical Practitioner who is to undertake the surgical procedure.

Information to enable informed consent

Information which is to be given to the patient who is to undergo surgical intervention, in order to assist him/her in giving informed consent, is best given by the Registered Medical Practitioner. This is a duty of care which the doctor owes to the patient. Generally speaking in the UK, nurses do not perform direct surgery, and therefore the duty of obtaining valid consent lies with the doctor. However, nurses have a responsibility to ensure that consent has been granted. When the patient is about to sign, or has signed, the consent form, it is the nurse's duty to ensure that the patient understands the nature of the procedure. If s/he is in any doubt as to the patient's level of understanding of the intended procedure, then the nurse must notify the patient's Registered Medical Practitioner and ensure that the information imparted is given in such a manner that the patient will understand the full implications.

The consent process does not begin and end at this point. This important process may have been instigated during consultation at the outpatient department or a pre-assessment clinic. Meredith (1993) suggests that it is during the outpatient appointment that implied rules of communication and participation are imparted to patients through the context and routines the service providers. Inherent in this process is the importance of forming a relationship with the patient which is one of trust. Unlike a ward situation, where the nurse has had a greater opportunity to get to know the patient and form a trusting relationship, the time limitations of out-patient visits and day surgery care are not as conducive to this. Therefore, the signing of the consent form in a day surgery setting may be an endorsement of the relationship previously developed in the outpatient department, and hence the implications for establishing such a relationship early on are very clear.

As mentioned above, the signing of the consent form is not the be all and end all of permission to operate. Patients, sometimes after signing the consent form (at either the assessment clinic or in the day surgery unit) prior to surgery, may have a change of mind, for a variety of reasons. In the case of a minor, refusal to undergo treatment (surgical intervention to be included here) is usually governed by the Court of Appeal. The Court of Appeal have powers through the Family Law Reform Act 1969 Section Eight, to provide consent contrary to the minor or minor's parent's or legal guardian's wishes. Such cases are few, but may be met in day surgery settings. Take, for example, the procedure of sterilization. This was performed on a mentally handicapped minor, but not before the case went before the courts, who approved of the procedure. From this test case, it was established that every case of sterilization performed on a minor should come before the courts. Any nurse working in a day surgery setting who feels that the intended procedure (whatever it may be, or if sanctioned by parents and the minor's Registered Medical Practitioner) is not in the best interests of a child, should make known any reservations to senior management. It may then be considered necessary for the circumstances to be reviewed and referred to the courts for a judgement.

> Any nurse working in a day surgery setting who feels that the intended procedure is not in the best interests of a child, should make known any reservations to senior management.

Once having signed the consent form, any patient (or nurse) who has reservations about the intended procedure has a right (and duty, in the case of the nurse) to withdraw consent. This can only be done if all aspects of the case have been explored and it is established that the correct information has been given. A basic principle of law is that an adult, mentally competent person has the right to refuse treatment (Dimond 1995). The nurse has a duty of care to ensure that the patient's wishes are respected and also, and equally important, to take all reasonable precautions to ensure that the patient has the appropriate information on which to make a decision.

Nurses should be aware that patients who have been given a prescribed premedication prior to surgery are in no fit state to give a valid consent. Therefore, if, for whatever reason, the gaining of consent has been omitted or overlooked until after such drugs have been administered, then the treatment (in this case surgery) may be delayed.

> Nurses should be aware that patients who have been given a prescribed premedication prior to surgery are in no fit state to give valid consent. If the gaining of consent has been omitted until after such drugs have been administered, then the surgery may be delayed.

Thinking time. There are many ethical dilemmas that busy practising day surgery nurses may face. The issues surrounding consent are important. This chapter has focused on the issue of informed consent in detail. Box 8.2 describes two scenarios that you may wish to consider and offer possible solutions for. It must be remembered that each case will be context dependent and the solution may well be difficult.

■ **BOX 8.2 Two scenarios to be considered**

1. The patient has been anaesthetized and it is discovered that the consent form has not been signed; the dilemma is: should the procedure go ahead?

2. The patient has undergone an operative procedure and it is discovered that the consent form has not been signed; what course of action may ensue?

Content of information to enable informed consent to be given

What information should be provided to enable the patient to make that important decision? In order to serve the best interests of the patient, and to avoid an action of negligence for a breach of duty of care, the patient must be given vital information about the possible side effects of the proposed surgical procedure, i.e. from the moment the premedication is administered to a safe discharge and return to as near a 'normal' lifestyle as possible. Indeed, one of the seven rights listed in the Patient's Charter (1991) is the right to be 'given a clear explanation of any treatment proposed, including risks and any alternatives, before [you] decide ...'. Deciding on the nature and extent of the information which should be imparted to the patient can be difficult. To highlight any possible dilemma, it is worth referring to a test case. In Sidaway v. Bethlem Royal Hospital Governors and Others (1985), Amy Sidaway underwent a surgical operation on her spinal column to relieve constant pain in her neck. Prior to consent, her surgeon discussed with her the possible side effects (to an extent) and outlined the procedure. He did not however, warn her of the possibility of damage to the spinal cord (risk of damage is small – less than 1%), which could result in her being severely disabled. During the operative procedure Mrs Sidaway's spinal cord was, in fact, damaged, and this resulted in a severe disability. Mrs Sidaway attempted to sue the surgeon, alleging that she was not given all the facts which would have enabled her to give informed consent to the operation. She lost her case in the court, the Court of Appeal and the House of Lords. It was deemed appropriate for the surgeon to withhold or not inform Mrs Sidaway of all aspects of the potential problems. This practice was considered acceptable by a group of responsible neurosurgeons, who, faced with the same incident, would have acted in the same manner. This then set a precedent on which other cases are judged.

This case highlights the problems which may be encountered when attempting to give information to patients and to act in their best interests prior to obtaining valid consent. Whilst the Sidaway case is related to consent and the role of surgeon, the same principles could apply to the nurse. According to Clark and Gournay in Schober and Hinchliff (1995) there is a skill to information giving and the nurse needs to select the facts which are relevant and most useful to the patient. The aim is to offer information which is congruent with current, approved practice and, most importantly, is relevant to the individual's specific needs. The information given should reflect current, research-based practice. The question still remains – just how much information should the nurse give the patient? This can only be answered when the nurse has fully assessed the patient's needs and adheres to approved practice, practice which would be considered appropriate by an ordinary skilled nurse. It is not possible, therefore, to be dogmatic in defining how much information is to be given, as this will be context dependent. Nurses in day surgery settings would be wise, however, to constantly remind themselves of the UKCC's opening comments in the Code of Professional Conduct (1992a): '... to act in such a manner as to safeguard ... serve ... justify and uphold...'.

It is important that nurses give a balanced account of the realities of the proposed intervention, not only to ensure that true consent has been gained but also to pre-empt any problems which may occur during the patient's stay or on discharge. By providing patients with appropriate information which, it is hoped, will result in patient empowerment, patients will be in a better position to make informed choices about their care. Then, and only then, can true informed consent have been gained.

CHILDREN'S RIGHTS

Currently, the UKCC is considering the implementation of new regulations regarding student nurses working in clinical areas with children. It is proposed that by 1997 a nurse in training, allocated to an area where children are being nursed, can only perform clinical duties if at least two Registered Sick Children's Nurses (RSCN) are on duty. Such a requirement may have implications for nurses in day surgery settings.

A proposed Children's Charter

Children (those under 16 years of age) and minors (those aged between 16 and 17 years of age) utilize a number of services in the day surgery setting, and it is likely that such numbers, with the continued improvements in technology, will increase. At the moment, the Department of Health is awaiting feedback from the various professions associated with the welfare of children in order to compile a Children's Charter. This charter should help day surgery nurses to address the specific needs of children attending day surgery settings.

The Children Act 1989

The Children Act (1989) endeavours to ensure that a number of principles concerned with the welfare of children are adhered to. These principles demand that nurses, when caring for children, should:

• work with parents to enable them to care for them to the best of their ability;
• ensure that when working with children they listen to each child, provide appropriate information and take account of the child's wishes and feelings;

- identify children in need and, where appropriate, refer to the social services, and cooperate with the social services department and educational department to meet the needs of the children.

Children undergoing day surgery procedures have similar rights to those of adults. Informed consent has been addressed above. Children have unique needs, and this is also evident in day surgery settings. It is important that the nurse caring for children in day surgery settings has an awareness of the child's beliefs about health and illness. Children vary in this respect, and the child's developmental stage will need to be considered if the care provided is to be effective and relevant.

As outlined by Kennedy (Chapter 6), the issue of health and health promotion regarding children will extend to include the whole family unit. Nurses must remember that care and treatment will have repercussions for all members of the family.

Working with parents

It has long been accepted that parents should be involved with the child's care as much as possible, in order to promote recovery and make the experience a positive one. Whilst this may be limited because of the short period of hospitalization associated with day surgery settings, a child's perceptions of hospitals and the people who work in them is likely to be influenced by early experience. In day surgery settings the child's parents are actively involved in the care of the child. The parents stay with the child for as much of the procedure as they wish to be involved in.

The important and complex issue of confidentiality and children must be addressed. If an adult does not want the nurse to impart any information about him/herself, the nurse has a duty to respect this request (with some notable exceptions; see Dimond 1995 for further debate regarding these notable exceptions). In the case of children this is somewhat different. It was the Gillick case in the 1980s which paved the way for confidential information about a child to be made available to parents. In this case, it concerned the prescription of the contraceptive pill to a girl under 16 years of age. This case may also have some bearing on day surgery settings. An example could be the case of a girl under 16 years of age attending the day surgery setting for a termination of pregnancy. If the child in the nurse's care requested that confidential information, i.e. the termination of pregnancy, should not be given to the parent, then for the nurse to comply with such a request could result in his/her facing legal proceedings.

> Complying with a child's request not to give information to the parent could result in a nurse's facing legal proceedings.

Respecting the rights of children

The rights of children in the day surgery setting must be respected in order to satisfy legal requirements related to the nurse's duty of care. Clear guidelines should be provided to nurses by management, in order that both patient and clinicians are protected.

DAY SURGERY NURSES AS PRESCRIBERS

In March 1992 legislation was granted Royal assent permitting some nurses

> Powers to prescribe a limited number of listed drugs are currently applicable only to District Nurses and Health Visitors, not to other practising nurses.

to prescribe a limited number of listed drugs. At present these limited prescribing powers are currently applicable *only* to District Nurses and Health Visitors. It is important to note that these powers are not extended to other practising nurses, and, until such a time, practising nurses must abide by local policy and The Code of Professional Conduct. In some instances, there may be protocols which have been set up to permit surgical nurses to prescribe (for example Picolax). Where this is the case, this is a tripartite arrangement – nurses, pharmacist and doctor – sanctioned by the employing authority. For a nurse to be competent and confident with this expanded role, when, and if, it materializes s/he must be conversant with the UKCC's documents The Scope of Professional Practice (1992b), The Standards for the Administration of Medicines (1992c) and the Code of Professional Conduct (1992a).

An important aspect identified by the Scope of Professional Practice is that nurses practise in areas which are constantly changing and in order to practise safely, their practice must be sensitive, relevant and responsive to the needs of individual patients. They must be prepared to adjust, where and when appropriate, to changing circumstances (UKCC 1992b).

The future – prescribing powers extended?

It is possible that, in the not too-distant future, prescribing powers may extend to nurses working in other clinical areas. If the nurse practising in the day surgery setting agrees to undertake (when legislation permits) the extended power of limited prescribing then s/he must also embrace the tenets and rules within The Scope of Professional Practice, The Code of Professional Conduct and The Standards for the Administration of Medicines. Furthermore, in order to be competent in such an extended role, the nurse must be familiar with the legal regulations affecting the administration of drugs, for example The Misuse of Drugs Act 1971, The Medicines Act 1978, The Poisons Act 1972 and the various EC regulations which may need to be applied.

The Scope of Professional Practice demands that certain principles form the basis for any decisions relating to the extended role, and this could also be relevant to the extended role of the nurse prescriber. An outline of the principles related to the Scope of Professional Practice is as follows. The nurse should ensure that:

1. his/her practice meets the needs and interests of patients
2. s/he develops skill and competence
3. s/he acknowledges his/her limitations
4. s/he does not compromise existing care
5. s/he accepts personal accountability
6. s/he avoids inappropriate delegation.

Applying the principles in the Scope of Professional Practice to nurse prescribing

The following need to take into account in applying the six principles in The Scope of Professional Practice to nurse prescribing.

1. Paramount to undertaking the role of the nurse prescriber should be an understanding that the nurse must ensure that the activities to be undertaken contribute to meeting the needs and interests of the patient.
2. Fundamental to these principles, the nurse must ensure that his/her knowledge base is up to date, and that the skills required to act as nurse prescriber, which may include skills related to various routes used to administer medicines, are thorough. This also stresses the need for the nurse to be competent and responsive. Hence, flexibility, underpinned by a sound knowledge base, is vital if the nurse is to act within the requirements of The Scope of Professional Practice, The Code of Professional Conduct, and ultimately the law.
3. In order for the nurse to act in a manner which will do the patient no harm s/he must acknowledge any limitations in his/her knowledge and skills. This clause goes further in that it demands that actions are taken to remedy any deficiencies in order to meet safety and efficiency standards. In the future, such a requirement will also be necessary to conform to the content of PREPP (UKCC 1994).
4. The general care of the patient must not be compromised or fragmented by accepting the role of nurse prescriber. The nurse must ensure that the requirements of the Council in the form of the Code are not compromised in any way. If this is the case, then the nurse must remedy the situation in the most appropriate way. Failure to do so may lead to a charge of misconduct, and the nurse may find himself/herself the subject of disciplinary proceedings before the UKCC's Professional Conduct Committee. The employing authority may also take disciplinary action, and the patient may instigate legal civil proceedings against the nurse.
5. This clause points out to the nurse that s/he is personally accountable directly or indirectly for all professional actions. Hence, the notion of accountability which is so prominent in The Code of Professional Conduct is also central to the Scope of Practice.
6. The nurse must make it clear that the person delegating the task must do so with respect to the wider interests of society. The task must not be delegated in order to provide a means to an end. S/he must refuse to accept any delegated task that s/he considers is inappropriate or may cause harm or damage to others.

In order to adhere to these basic principles Dimond (1995) suggests that practitioners should have particular concerns which, when addressed, would include the following questions.

1. How do I know if I am competent?
2. How does my employer know if I am competent?
3. What happens if I undertake an activity outside my field of competence?
4. Where do I stand if a doctor/senior manager/other professional ignores my refusal to undertake an activity because I do not have sufficient competence or experience to undertake this activity?

The nurse must satisfy her/himself that s/he is competent to undertake the procedure and, if incompetent, must make this lack of competence known to the person delegating the task. No nurse is permitted to undertake any task which falls outside his/her sphere of competence and skill. A fundamental tenet of the Code of Professional Conduct requires nurses to acknowledge any limitations in knowledge and competence. The nurse therefore needs to examine his/her capabilities and decline to undertake any duty which s/he may feel that s/he is not capable of performing. There are certain contractual considerations which the nurse will be able to fulfil prior to undertaking duties required for the post which s/he holds. A nurse can refuse to undertake an activity because of insufficient knowledge, expertise or competence. It is unacceptable to plead the case 'I was carrying out orders'.

> The nurse must satisfy her/himself that s/he is competent to undertake a procedure and, if incompetent, must make this lack of competence known to the person delegating the task. A nurse can refuse to undertake an activity because of insufficient knowledge, expertise or competence.

Whilst the above discussion is primarily concerned with the contents of the document entitled The Scope of Professional Practice, it also encroaches on, and indeed is verified by, several other important supplementary documents issued by the UKCC. These were referred to at the beginning of the chapter.

The notion of nurses (in all care settings) being granted limited prescribing powers may not be far off, and the principles outlined may equally apply to nurses in day surgery settings.

This chapter began by discussing the ethical and moral schools of thought and ends by asking nurses in day surgery settings to consider these schools of thought and the Professional Codes and Guidelines when attempting to make complex clinical decisions regarding informed consent, children's rights and the possibility of day surgery nurses being granted limited prescribing powers.

DOCUMENTATION OF CARE

> Nurses must be aware that nursing documents are potential legal documents.

It is vital that the care delivered to the patient in the day surgery setting is documented. Careful documentation of care will be required if the nurse is asked to demonstrate that there was no negligence relating to the care given. Nursing documents are not legal documents. However, the nurse must be made aware of the fact that they are potential legal documents (Young 1991).

What constitutes nursing notes?

A variety of documents used by nurses could be considered to be nursing notes. Nurses also use other documents to record incidents – accident books, prescription charts and the controlled drugs register, for example. By far the first and most obvious document is the nursing care plan. Details on this document will enable the reader to ascertain each stage of the nursing process assessments, planned care, the way in which it was implemented and the results of that intervention – the evaluation. The content of these stages of the nursing process may have legal implications, if the patient wishes to plead that the nurse(s) was/were negligent when caring for him/her at any stage of his/her stay in the day surgery unit. As many day surgery nurses also scrub and assist with operative procedures within the day surgery unit, this can have far-reaching implications. Elsewhere in this text Phelan and Grenside discuss the role of the day surgery theatre nurse. Documentation of care and the contents of the care plans may also be used in audit. Fearon (Chapter 10) discusses quality and audit issues further.

The correct, thorough and careful documentation of care in a busy, high-turnover area such as a day surgery unit can only lead to improved communication, a reduction in mishaps and an enhancement of continuity of care (see Hodge, Chapter 7). Documentation of care is one of two forms of communication. Firstly, there is verbal communication in the handover of patient from unit nurse to anaesthetic nurse, anaesthetic nurse to scrub nurse, scrub nurse to recovery nurse and recovery nurse to unit nurse. The purpose of these communications is to ensure that a current, comprehensive, accurate and concise report concerning the patient's condition and the care received is provided in order to promote safety and efficiency and aid the patient's recovery (UKCC 1993, Murdock 1995). Secondly, there is the written account of what has been done and the proposed plan of care.

Documentation of care is an important task, and has been seen as a problematic issue in the past. The Department of Health and the UKCC therefore deemed it necessary to publish two important documents to help health care professionals with their record keeping (Department of Health 1992, UKCC 1993).

A variety of initiatives have also recently been introduced which demand that health care records are maintained in order to enhance patient care. For example, The Patient's Charter (1991), The Data Protection Act (1984), and The Access to Health Care Records Act (1990) are all relevant when considering record and document keeping.

The Data Protection Act and The Access to Medical Records Act

The Data Protection Act allows patients legal access to computerized medical records. The patient is able to gain access to his/her records for a small fee and has the right to rectify any misrepresentations made in the data base (Dimond 1995). However, there are some restrictions. The right of access can be denied if the person is likely to suffer either physical or mental injury from the content of the record. Only certain listed, appropriate health care professions have the right to this exercise in disclosure, and, in some circumstances, this may apply to the Registered Nurse.

> Patients have a legal right to access their medical records. Access can be denied, however, if the patient is likely to suffer physical or mental injury from the content of the record. Access to manual records made before 1 November 1991 can be denied.

This Act, it must be emphasized, relates only to materials held on computer. It could be suggested that if information technology continues to increase and expand at its current rate, this will have further implications for day surgery nurses, who may find most of their documentation of care confined to computerized records.

Manual records are protected by The Access to Medical Records Act (1991). It is important to note that this Act was effective from 1 November 1991 and is not retrospective. This means that should an individual require details from records made earlier than 1 November 1991, access can be denied. Again, under The Access to Medical Records Act, exemptions to access can also apply and they are similar to the exemptions discussed in relation to The Data Protection Act (1984).

Who contributes to the nursing notes?

The UKCC (1993) has recognized the advantages of shared record keeping and suggests that the best way forward is to agree to the formation of a local policy for guidance, as long as this has the best interests of the patient as its central focus.

In day surgery settings the approach to nursing documentation is often a multidisciplinary nurse-led approach. The skilled nurse carries out an in-depth psychological, physical and social assessment and then makes referrals to other members of the multidisciplinary team with regard to any problems that are outside their competence. For example, an in-depth preanaesthetic assessment is undertaken by the nurse, and, if required, an anaesthetist's opinion is requested. The accountable nurse then completes the preoperative check list. Perioperative documentation is then completed by the scrub nurse. The anaesthetist records and documents the intra-operative physiological condition of the patient and gives any specific postoperative instructions. The nurse accountable for the discharge process also documents this important information. Different types of documentation may exist for different procedures, e.g. intravenous sedation, or different client groups, e.g. children.

Standards for records and record keeping

The UKCC (1993) produced the standards document after growing concern emerged concerning poor documentation which could suggest poor care which may, in turn, result in negligence. Indeed, Castledine (1993) suggests that with respect to quality, accountability and documentation of care, nurses are performing at a below average level. The UKCC (1993) lists four areas where there are problems associated with documentation of care:

- continuity of care
- communication between staff
- the risk of medication and communication being duplicated
- failure to focus attention on early signs of deviation from the norm
- failure to place on record significant observations and conclusions.

Prior to these concerns being expressed by the UKCC, The Audit Commission (1991) also voiced concern and suggested that nurses must make more comprehensive nursing notes in order to enhance and improve the quality of care.

Key factors in documenting care

It is important that documentation of an episode is done as soon as possible after the event has occurred, in order to accurately reflect the incident. The record should include details which are readily understood by all who have access to the documentation. The person who completes the record must write in terms which are unambiguous and clear. The entry made by the day surgery nurse must be totally accurate, honest and legible; s/he must write in indelible black ink (to facilitate photocopying), not pencil. A date and time must accompany each entry. It is unacceptable to use correcting fluid to make any amendment to an entry. One single line through the section to be deleted is sufficient. This must also be signed and dated. Abbreviations must be avoided. If they are used, one interpretation of the abbreviated word must be agreed upon by all staff in order to avoid confusion and ultimately harm.

> Records should be completed in good time and should be unambiguous, clear, accurate, honest and legible. Correcting fluid should not be used to make an amendment; a single line through the section to be deleted is sufficient. Date and time must accompany each entry.

The aim in documenting nursing care is to serve the best interests of the patient, promote care, prevent disease and promote health (UKCC 1993). Furthermore, the record will demonstrate where, when, why and what happened. It could be suggested that if it was not documented then it was not done, and if it was not described, then it was not seen.

CONCLUSION

The most important question any nurse in the day surgery setting must ask when considering all options must be 'Am I acting within my sphere of competence and will my actions be in the best interests of the patient?'

REFERENCES

Audit Commission 1991 The virtue of patients: making the best use of nursing resources. HMSO, London
Castledine G 1993 Can performance related pay be adapted for nursing? British Journal of Nursing 2(22): 1120–1121
Clark E, Gournay K 1995 The individual and health. In: Schober J E, Hinchliff H (eds) Towards advanced nursing practice. Arnold, London
Department of Health 1991 The Patient's Charter. HMSO, London
Department of Health 1992 Nursing records. Circular PL/CNO (92) 10. HMSO, London
Dimond B 1995 Legal aspects of nursing, 2nd edn. Prentice Hall, London
Great Britain, Parliament 1969 The Family Reform Act. HMSO, London
Great Britain, Parliament 1971 The Misuse of Drugs Act. HMSO, London
Great Britain, Parliament 1972 The Poisons Act. HMSO, London
Great Britain, Parliament 1978 The Medicines Act. HMSO, London
Great Britain, Parliament 1983 The Mental Health Act. HMSO, London
Great Britain, Parliament 1984 The Data Protection Act. HMSO, London
Great Britain, Parliament 1989 The Children Act. HMSO, London
Great Britain, Parliament 1990 The Access to Health Care Records Act. HMSO, London
Meredith P 1993 Patient participation in decision making and consent to treatment: the case of surgery. Sociology of Health and Illness 15(3): 315–335
Murdock D 1995 Careful recording. Nursing Times 91(47): 44–45
Sidaway v. Bethlem Royal Hospital Governors and Others 1985 1 All ER 643
Thiroux J 1980 Ethics, theory and practice, 2nd edn. Glencoe Publishing, California
Tschundin V 1992 Ethics in nursing – the caring relationship. Heinemann, Oxford
United Kingdom Central Council 1987 Confidentiality. UKCC, London
United Kingdom Central Council 1992a Code of professional conduct. UKCC, London
United Kingdom Central Council 1992b Scope of professional practice. UKCC, London
United Kingdom Central Council 1992c Standards for the administration of medicines. UKCC, London
United Kingdom Central Council 1993 Standards for records and record keeping. UKCC, London
United Kingdom Central Council 1994 The future of professional practice: the Council's standards for education and practice following registration. UKCC, London
Young P 1991 Law and professional conduct in nursing. Scutari Press, London

Research and day surgery practice

Louise Gamble

The human faculties of perception, judgement, discriminative feeling, mental acuity and even moral preference are exercised only in making a choice. He who does anything because it is the custom makes no choice. He gains no practice either in discerning or desiring what is best. The mental and moral, like the muscular powers, are improved only by being used.

(John Stuart Mill, On Liberty, 1859)

Research is vital. It derives its energy from its dynamic pursuit to capture and reflect meaning and understanding. The quest to identify, describe and give credence to the concepts, practice, context and outcomes of nursing occupies nurse researchers with increasing dedication and momentum as they strive to shape the profession's professional purpose. Increasingly, nursing is being called to account, and the principles and virtues of its practice must be established for its continued value to the individual and society to be sustained.

INTRODUCTION

The purpose of this chapter is to indicate the role of research in the pursuit of nursing excellence. Involvement in research can occur at different levels, and the opportunities available afford all nurses the chance to participate. Justice cannot be done within the limitations of this chapter to the detail of research, but an overview of the elements that contribute towards its production and utilization will be outlined. The challenge to utilize research findings and the opportunity to conduct research studies, within the context of day surgery, form the two main themes of this chapter. A particularly important feature in this chapter is the significance of all nurses becoming consumers and users of research whilst at the same time realizing that not all will become nurse researchers.

Despite these worthy notions, supported by an increasing volume of research publications, there still seems to be a certain reluctance to become involved in the generation, participation, implementation or evaluation of research findings. To acknowledge the value and purpose of research without reference to the reality of some of the difficulties associated with its generation and application would be to deny research its potential influence. However well-intentioned the motivation and desire to become involved in research, there are certain barriers to be overcome. The deliberate exposure of these barriers may breach their resistance as they are rendered vulnerable by this scrutiny. Indeed barriers must not be allowed to form exclusion zones, but if viewed as the frontiers to be explored and extended they may draw the attention of researchers.

The negative potential of turning day surgery into an automated, predetermined service of rationed procedures controlled by bureaucratic documentation systems must be avoided. The largely non-residential nature of day surgery should never be allowed to undermine the status and needs of the patient. The particular challenges of day surgery, often reflected in the brevity and pace of the nurse–patient encounter, should establish the positive potential to initiate nursing research studies. The challenge in day surgery is to manage and streamline patient care in a professional, collaborative, high-quality and cost-effective manner enhanced by the opportunity to conduct research and utilize appropriate findings and recommendations.

A Strategic Research Matrix is suggested to represent some of those resources and skills concerned with implementing research and sustaining the momentum of learning. The matrix is ultimately patient-focused and depends on the effort of nursing practitioners, educators and managers to access and select information that is relevant, valid and credible. The resultant usefulness of research-based nursing should inform and reflect significant aspects of professional purpose and practice. There is a variety of ways in which knowledge, learning and experience can be acquired and developed. Together with the more intuitive and aesthetic ways of knowing, less amenable to evidence-based theory, research ought to culminate in the nursing wisdom that establishes its intrinsic value for the individual, family and society.

RESEARCH, AUDIT AND CURIOSITY

It is important to distinguish research and audit in health care as the interface between them may become blurred. Research aims to identify and establish optimal treatment, practice and care, and it explores or discovers new endeavours through which it compares performance against agreed standards or criteria. Audit is an ongoing process within a specific or designated area of examination and incorporates the participants' input. The findings are consistently channelled back into practice to effect the necessary change as indicated by audit convention (Thomson Report 1993). Audit relies on the principled integrity of the current practice and does not attempt to question its inherent authenticity. It might be argued that using audit to measure patient outcomes is unwise unless research demonstrates clearly that patients have improved as a direct result of their treatment and care. Attributing improvements through audit studies should be avoided until research establishes the credibility and validity of the audited differentials. If a day surgery unit is to consider using audit as a qualitative measure or an agent for change, then responsibility must be taken to confirm the research base of the audit focus.

Research findings may be extrapolated beyond the population or focus of study, as quantitative research relies on sampling and controls to produce results that can be generalized and replicated. The end-point of research does not always implicate change as a natural corollary, whereas audit results are considered as indications for change. Research is more frequently published in journals whose main purpose is to disseminate information and promote education. Unlike audit, in which change is integral, research does not require a structured method to implement its results. However, this is not entirely unreasonable, as many research studies involve new evidence, contain methodological bias and may ultimately depend on the researcher's technique. The implementation of research may also depend on the ability to appraise the methodology and on the skill to innovate change.

Research and audit can be compared and distinguished by their contrasting methods of discovery in the formation of knowledge (Nolan & Behi 1995). However, there are other ways of seeking and acquiring knowledge that are considered part of our natural, everyday curiosity and experience. Influential beliefs and perceptions can affect judgement and reasoning and must function along with and not to the exclusion of systematic enquiry and analysis. Satisfying our natural human curiosity about the world around us sustains our motivation, promotes examination of our drives and shapes our reality. Indeed formalizing our intellectual and emotional endeavours through research methodologies and methods may be a more natural enterprise than at first recognized. Perhaps research is the 'Fourth R'? The arousal of this state of curiosity has the potential of developing a positive attitude towards research (Figure 9.1).

THE ROLE OF RESEARCH

To encapsulate the world of research within a single definition is of little value except to note that most distinguish its specific role as being to discover, produce and present knowledge in a systematic and scientific manner (Nolan & Behi 1995). However, to continually demonstrate evidence without recourse to its applied relevance would serve only to widen the so called theory–practice gap (Rolfe 1996). The status of becoming a nurse researcher in comparison with the utility of being a consumer and user of research has perhaps contributed to the exclusion of many research findings from past and current nursing practice. Concentration on the methodologies and methods of research has taken precedence over the development of critical appraisal and practical implementation. The subject of research can be taught and evaluated within a classroom setting, but it is much more complicated to assure its practical utilization and assessment following its achievement. The hidden agenda of research commonly existing as a feature of an educational course or a programme hoop to be jumped though may contribute towards its apparent theoretical inclusion and practical exclusion. In this climate the utilization of research

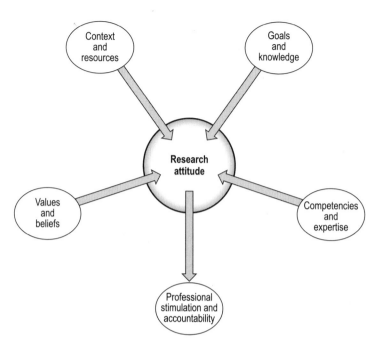

Figure 9.1 The fundamental components influencing a positive research attitude. Adapted from Deane & Campbell (1985).

becomes an organizational and attitudinal problem rather than a professional nursing priority. The apparent difficulties in selecting and implementing relevant research-based evidence in an atmosphere of indifference and secondary ignorance (i.e. an individual cannot know what they do not know) produce an environment that implicitly resists and denies the value of research. Any definition should therefore contain not only the theoretical substances of research but indeed the potential and manner of its implementation.

The primary purpose of nursing research is to develop and advance nursing knowledge. If implemented successfully it should make a critical difference to patient outcomes and guide what education is most appropriate for nursing. Nursing knowledge therefore gains verification and ensures professional survival (Treece & Treece 1986). By providing new approaches for flexibility and individual choice, it prevents obsolescence, indicates the need for accelerated change and provides direction for individual renewal. It may also prove nursing's capability to respond in today's society with a collective professional identity. The increased prestige of conducting and implementing research is well recognized in higher education establishments, with which many traditional colleges and schools of nursing have now merged, and has a status which is historically proven, valued and respected within these institutions.

Research is a method of obtaining knowledge through organized scientific and systematic enquiry (Treece & Treece 1986), the findings of which are the product and result of the specific research methodology used. This considered approach distinguishes research from the unstructured knowledge acquired from experience or intuition. However, it can be argued that there are qualitative research processes that may uncover the nuances and intricacies of unique humanistic events that do not lend themselves easily to quantitative scientific scrutiny. The purpose of nursing research should be to increase the understanding of nursing practice in order to positively affect direct patient care. This is achieved by its unifying influence on education, practice and management. Nurse educators are obligated not just to deliver information as substance, but also to use it as a learning medium that will bring about a healthy and balanced scepticism. It is the development of this curiosity that has the potential of bringing about research-mindedness. By generating knowledge that confirms and increases the integrity of the nursing curriculum and work-based setting and enriches what might be described as nursing's intuitive or tacit humanistic qualities, e.g. compassion, gentleness, kindness, concern, research lays claim to nursing for nurses.

Within the brevity of the day surgery encounter it might be too easy for individuals who know no different, to presume that if adequate training could be given to non-nursing ancillary staff the entire process could be driven by instrumental convention and intent rather than by nurses empowered through their knowledge base, collegiality and professional vocational purpose. The burgeoning development of day surgery has been, and must continue to be, a remarkable opportunity to clarify and articulate nursing benefits into patient outcomes. Research provides the opportunity to defend nursing's role through the testing and evaluation implicit within the exercise of enquiry. The credibility and validity of research findings are powerful prerequisites for initiating change. They underline the professional responsibility to ensure that the best options are available. Without research how does nursing judge the effectiveness of practice? Audit relies on standards derived from research, and it would be unethical to base audit on unconfirmed or dubious practice. This specific need for research-based knowledge answers the frequent criticism that it only tells us what we already know. As indicated earlier, research often explores or discovers novel information, thus raising new questions, increasing levels of awareness and promoting further study.

It would be unreasonable for nurses to rely entirely on their individual reasoning and judgement, ignoring research evidence, and claim to be professional in their practice. The gravity of health care needs is too great for them to be treated in such a cavalier fashion. Research alerts us to undesirable circumstances and, through its predictive qualities, guides us towards enticing goals. Research has a responsibility, if it is to be relevant to practice, to make some of today's health care encounters less uncertain, unstable, incomplete and complex by revealing alternative options that positively affect direct patient care. Informed consent is an issue that nursing regards as imperative for patients, and it is no less important that nurses choose to consent in an informed manner to practice nursing. The implications within the law, professional codes and local health policies related to accountability should concentrate the research-mindedness of the nursing profession to ensure that conduct and use of research become the integral themes that drive nursing excellence and clinical effectiveness.

Research into health and nursing issues is paramount in respect of the gravity of illness for the individual, family and society. Research findings should influence prioritization within strategic health policy and planning and impact upon decision-making, but at present nursing research appears to have little influence compared with that of the medical profession (Closs & Cheater 1995). Nursing is a distinct and significant part of health care delivery and it must demonstrate its influence and value. The establishment of a confirmed body of knowledge is a fundamental characteristic of a profession, reflecting its unity and level of empowerment.

The repercussions of published research evidence can marshal and accelerate support from those who are responsible for providing vital resources. Risks can be identified and responded to, and accessibility of effective health resources can be more easily sustained. Research is a planned and balanced response to an area of doubt or concern, and therefore its results should produce a much clearer range of options in the best interests of patient care.

Historically, nursing was well known for its traditional task-bound tactics and organization strengthened by the fragmented presence of a largely transient workforce. Through the potent and energetic drive of nursing research there is now a real opportunity to establish distinctive roles, competencies, effective leadership and collaborative practice. Providing new approaches and deeper understanding engenders flexibility and individual choice. It prevents obsolescence, indicates the need for change and provides direction for renewal. Research has the potential to reactivate latent expertise and commitment extinguished by indifferent practice. It is not enough just to learn nursing – today it is more important to learn how to be effective as a nurse. It is skilled and effective application of constructed knowledge that distinguishes the educated expert from the limitations of the procedure-bound novice. Nursing is being called to account, and, as failure does not go unnoticed, nursing practice needs defence and justification or it may become disempowered.

BARRIERS AND CONSTRAINTS

Despite the established value of research and its contribution to the body of nursing knowledge, it has generally failed to influence practice in a substantial manner (English 1994). Nursing remains undecided about its nature and purpose. The perception of the status of nursing remains low, and its struggle to identify its professional and unique function is confounded by the difficulty of isolating nursing practice from the collaborative contribution to patient care by other health professionals. Nursing research is a much smaller endeavour in relation to similar vocations (e.g. medicine), and as nursing research is also less established as a tradition it lacks the influential immediacy of medicine's material weight, credibility, impetus and significance (Mulhall 1995). The substantiated predominance of health policy and planning related to medical enterprise and research masks the potential and prioritization of nursing research. The funding and support for research within higher education can be a source of conflict for traditional and established faculties. Nursing, as one of the most recent to join, may not yet have developed the track-record or strategies to compete for parity in such funding. Health care policy planners may not even be aware of the role, purpose and potential of nursing to affect patient outcomes. Even within health care organizations, does the management structure recognize the value of nursing in terms of established or potential nursing research? Predetermined clinical demands can be manipulated to distinguish approximate levels of funding, whereas the infinite demands of patient needs are less susceptible to predictable funding establishment. The direct nursing patient care policy and planning is minimal, fragile and inconsistent. Nursing has a moral imperative to ensure that health care is determined by providing a service that addresses needs, alternatives and choice. Maintaining a patient-centred focus may prevent health care from becoming a predetermined ration of restricted offers. Nursing research must respond to both practice and policy. However, the dilemmas that exist between the form of nursing that is encapsulated within our professional codes and the terms of our employment, which more frequently dictate what we do rather than how we do it, distinguish some of the barriers and constraints of the influential forms of governance.

The rapidity of change has gained precedence over the content of change, which can blur or prevent the identification and generation of potential research. Unless a definitive strategy for nursing research can be established at national and local levels to reflect organizational goals, professional and educational development cannot make progress effectively. The preferential position of being in control of change rather than the unsolicited recipient of it forms a considerable part of the perceived role of the present and future graduate nurse. Traditionally the professional has accepted delegated tasks, roles and received knowledge as pragmatic compliance within a hierarchical and patriarchal system of governance. Today's emphasis on empowerment and self-determination should increase the uptake of, and involvement with, research.

A further dilemma arises from the pursuit of nursing knowledge. It may appear a worthy and empowering activity, but as well as distinguishing strengths it may also indicate weaknesses and insecurity. The avoidance of involvement in research activities masks the vulnerability of nursing and relegates the threat of the traditional status quo's being challenged. The avoidance of conflict and dissonance also sustains this status quo. A healthy scepticism of tradition and current practice must be generated to prevent indifference, protectionism and stasis. If nursing only becomes galvanized into active research by accident or fear of litigation then the profession will be unable to retain respect, influence or value.

A research culture and environment should not be seen as entirely separate from other educational initiatives. Career pathways must be matched by sensitive education pathways and opportunities. Valuing clinical practice in equal weight to theoretical achievement is vital. Educational strategies to promote critical thinking, decision-making, problem-solving and evaluation skills must form the mainstay of the educational process. The theory–practice gap could be more readily approximated if research were derived from the contextual reality of practice. Research might also be viewed more advantageously if clinical examples were more easily demonstrated as successes.

Research has grown in the shadow of 'ivory towers', the academic purpose of research being seen as furnishing individual goals rather than enhancing the collective professional purpose of nursing. As the professional purpose of research may be more specifically identified by nurse researchers who are action or clinically oriented, they should be encouraged to focus their research according to an articulate clinical purpose in respect of contextual reality. The academic researcher may not achieve clinical practicality since, although motivated by other equally valid purposes, s/he may be unable to distinguish the subtleties, nuances, and intricacies and realities of nursing experience.

Many research studies are pursued as part of educational development and not directly addressed to clinical needs. Thus research as a fertile means to an impotent end may be viewed as a sterile endeavour. Staff development programmes will cease to participate with and in continuing education if the research and learning gained is not influencing practice. Reorganization of traditional clinical pathways (e.g. day surgery) and community reconfiguration will cause a revision of nursing. A consortium of educational, clinical and managerial interests to generate, nurture and appraise nursing research could create the climate that will ensure the best interests of the patient, profession and organization are in safe hands.

These barriers and constraints reveal only some of the clinical, managerial and educational concerns that restrict the conduct and use of research. Perhaps a persistent limitation is the apparent unshakeable belief in ourselves as embryonic nurses, already accomplished in humanitarian skills before we applied to commence our preregistration education, the presence of the curriculum regarded only as a necessary hurdle rather than an enriching experience to transform our personal skills into therapeutic nursing qualities?

RESEARCH APPROACHES

Nursing research is a systematic endeavour and method to achieve solutions within the domain of nursing through the collection of quantitative and qualitative information for the professional purpose of prediction and exploration. While quantitative research measures discrete knowledge, qualitative research explores broad concerns related to human experience, generating a rich descriptive knowledge base. Whatever the planned or tentative examination of facts, meanings or relationships through which research is performed, the pursuit of excellence is a worthy challenge (LoBiondo-Wood & Haber 1994).

The form of research inquiry may also imply the type of knowledge likely to be discovered. Basic research can reveal knowledge, from a scientific methodology, in its own right without necessarily indicating a specific application. Applied research can be purposeful and focused on distinct practical objectives. It may be said that research can either generate new knowledge or improved knowledge. Applied research into the improvement of gaslight may have enhanced methods of gas illumination but it would not necessarily have led to the discovery of electric light. Indeed this comparison ought to emphasize the need for both forms (basic and applied) of research in nursing. Day surgery not only demands improvement and adaptation of current nursing skills but it also needs basic research to define its value as an innovative totality in its own right.

Accepting the need for, and potential of, research to advance nursing practice, and having paid respect to some of the educational, practice-based and managerial barriers to be overcome or avoided, enables the embryonic researcher to examine the various approaches and methods available. This examination may be guided by the nature of the research question as to whether a qualitative or quantitative approach would elicit reliable, valid and/or credible evidence. These two approaches contrast the differential aspects of the objective physical world (quantitative) or the subjective social existence. When Pythagorus discovered 'his' theory it had already existed independently since time immemorial (quantitative) unaffected by events, people or climate. However studies of moral behaviour or the concept of patient comfort may be influenced by circumstances, time or emotions (qualitative) demonstrating the dependent existence of meaning as a conscious and subjective observation (LoBiondo-Wood & Haber 1994).

The broad principles underlying the approaches to quantitative and qualitative methodology are illustrated inTable 9.1. Historically, quantitative scientific research has maintained an academic dominance due largely to its inherent ability to rely on consistency and the reliable cause-and-effect laws of universality. Reliability reflects the extent to which a specified factor yields consistent information indicating stability, accuracy and dependability (Treece & Treece 1986). It can be seen to be trustworthy, and therefore people can invest their commitment to it. This approach and associated methodologies constitute a legitimate manner in which to proceed if the subjectivity of contextual realities is of little significance.

If the quantitative approach is applied to individuals or societies, it is of concern that the subjective integrity of relationships and meaningful observations will not emerge. Just as there are a number of ways in which quantitative research may be implemented, so too are there numerous approaches to qualitative research. Despite the two contrasting methodologies which underpin the nature of the researchable focus, both can share the same methods of eliciting data (e.g. questionnaires and observation). Both share the necessity to demonstrate and discuss their findings and, if appropriate, make conclusions and give recommendations. The opportunity to describe the particular nature and strategies of research methodology is outwith the remit of this chapter, and further detail will be obtained in the recommended reading suggested.

In nursing there is no particular influence as to which methodology is more likely to produce clinical effectiveness. However, it is essential that nurse researchers pursue questions worthy of examination and endeavour to influence practice by indicating the routes for effective implementation of significant findings. It has been noted that many famous researchers are remembered for the generation of the researchable question rather than the conduct of the study. Involvement in research is perhaps somewhat

Table 9.1 A comparison of the broad principles of quantitative and qualitative methodologies

Quantitative	Qualitative
Approach: Logical empiricism Positivism Scientific–experimental Survey	*Approach*: Critical social theory Grounded theory Ethnography Phenomenology
Focus: Concise, narrow, reductionist, objective, exclusive, fixed	*Focus*: Complex, broad, holistic, subjective, inclusive, variable, natural
Reasoning: Logical, deductive, exclusive of researcher bias	*Reasoning*: Dialectic, inductive and shared meaning Influence may exist between researcher and study groups
Ways of knowing: Cause/effect relationships, tests theories, control, pilot studies, instruments ∴ manipulative irrespective of time and place	*Ways of knowing*: Meaning, discovery, develops theory, atheoretical, communication, observation ∴ inclusive of contextual reality and tacit knowledge
Elements of analysis: Numbers, statistical analysis, measurement of hard data	*Elements of analysis*: Words, individual interpretation, contextual, judgement
Findings: Generalization Reliability and validity	*Findings*: Unique Credible and verified

daunting at first, and the suggestion that 'action research' may be a gentler introduction should be addressed.

ACTION RESEARCH

'Action research' relates to an approach which appears to fuse problem-solving, implementation and evaluation in a single process of conducting research and using results implicit in audit systems. It offers the freedom of an eclectic choice of methodology and method that may be more likely to approximate the dissonance between nursing theory and its application. Within this divide lie the unpredictable, uncertain, incomplete, atypical and multifaceted circumstances in which nursing practice takes place. It is suggested that it is these contextual variables that sustain the dichotomy rather than any gross inherent fault in the ideology of the theory of the reality of the practice. Action research appears to account for this by inviting the naturally occurring humanity and context of unique situations to be taken into consideration when attempting to resolve problems.

In comparison with either the academic pursuit or the centralized commissioning of nursing research, action research appears to be less dependent on large funding requests or professional researchers and therefore offers a degree of independence and focus for individual renewal and empowerment. Nursing is now so concentrated and complex that a spiral model of collaborative research based on a rational participatory democracy within the profession is needed. This may relegate the legacy of suspicion surrounding research and ensure that its implementation is relevant to accurately assessed requirements. Action research is a spiral, rather than linear model, involving the interchanging roles of researcher, disseminator and practitioner, which underpins the value of people rather than processes (methodology). Both quantitative and qualitative methodology have faults related to the objective/prescriptive and subjective/descriptive outcomes of each (Webb 1989).

Recalling the previous brief descriptions of quantitative and qualitative research which depend on single approaches and their manner of exploiting the subject material, action researchers find the open and participative nature of 'critical science' specifically attractive and sensitive to issues in nursing research. The emergence of critical science, which establishes the autonomy and responsibility of participants, can be used by action researchers and offers a broader theoretical outcome through its contextual interpretation, implicit and explicit value systems, and the individuality of the participants involved. Its form could almost be compared with the need and scope of informed consent. The knowledge developed from the new theory is grounded in actual and current practice, attributes and limitations of the local circumstances. In this manner the action researcher, for instance the nursing practitioner, becomes not just a knowledgeable agent but indeed a knowledge maker and user.

The linear process of traditional research method contrasts with the spiral model of action research (Figure 9.2). The primary or preliminary recognition of a problem or issue worthy of exploration is identified in Stages 1 and 2. The research methodology is then determined by an action plan, Stages 2–4, which clarifies the issues and options for scrutiny, including resources, personnel, ethics, limitations and strengths established by a literature search and review. At this point the action researcher may wish to implement the verification implied in the use of triangulation studies. Triangulation involves more than a single research method to determine the authenticity and reflexivity of a critical-science methodology. Reflexivity (Webb 1991) relates to the openness and honesty of the action researcher, using critical science, to ensure that any deviation, bias or personal implications are detailed as part of the research process. Stages 5 and 6 form the innovatory process of action research. The monitoring and evaluation of the reconfigured or changed focus of the research study will elicit the verification of the findings from Stages 4 and 5. However the spiral nature of action research continues at the secondary reflection at Stage 7 through the ongoing readjustment of further action research and potential improvement.

Cohen & Manion (1985) characterize action research as *situational* (contextual), *collaborative* (spiral interaction), *participatory* (implementation of findings) and *self-evaluative*, emphasizing its central focus of improving practice. There is a growing movement in favour of action research, despite the continuing debate on the effectiveness of diverse research method-

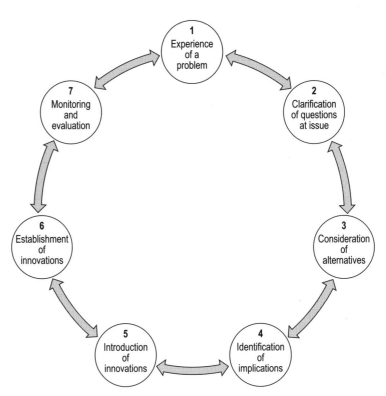

Figure 9.2 The continuous and reflective spiral nature of 'action research'. Adapted from Webb (1991).

ologies and the difficulty in structuring a problem to suit research scrutiny and dissemination of findings (Greenwood 1994).

RESEARCH INVOLVEMENT AND UTILIZATION

Using the word RE-SE-AR-CH, the author has developed a Strategic Research Matrix to facilitate a non-threatening and progressively staged research involvement (Figure 9.3). The matrix is an attempt to encapsulate the major aspects of research involvement in a sequential and continuous loop. The structural aspects of motivating and supporting the necessity to read and select require the active resourcing of learning from management, education and the individual nurse. The processes of critical thinking and analysis (Rubenfeld & Scheffer 1995) are the result of the measured exploration of concepts, facts, principles, assumptions and values. The first consideration in starting to read, in this productive manner, is finding the time without interruption, to concentrate and think. Critical reading skills should enable the development of a deep understanding of the significant issues involved and their consequential relationships. Material to read, in the first instance can be selected from a variety of resources. Sheehan (1994) discusses the value of journal clubs as influential resources for education and learning, as more appropriate guidance and focus may be determined by its members.

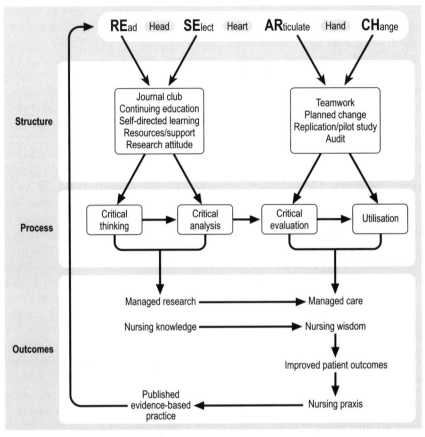

Figure 9.3 Nursing RE-SE-AR-CH: stages and processes of research utilization suggesting the reflective route from practice to research to theory to practice (Praxis).

Deliberate selection of particular and related subject matter concentrates effort. If research is to be examined in a purposeful manner as the outcome to generate enhanced nursing knowledge, a specific literature search and review requires good and selective management. Indeed the initial skill of reading may rest on the ability to select from an overwhelming choice. New understanding may entail destabilization of previously-held notions and principles, and this may be difficult to accept. This may be particularly true if it also conflicts with current practice. In effect, critical thinking through practised reading skills is the first step towards the selective ability of analysis and evaluation.

Waiting for the next edition of the journal to arrive may provide relevant material by chance. Selecting the broad topic areas through specialist journals or texts is more likely to provide relevant material. Deliberate selection of particular and related subject matter focuses attention and concentrates effort. There is little excuse today for being unable to collect resources for study, as nursing and public libraries, the media and information technology offer a remarkable choice. Choice may also depend on the personal bias and knowledge base of the reader. Reading and thinking also require an emotional as well as an intellectual commitment to concentrate. If the motivation of channelling nursing practice towards enhanced patient outcomes is to be satisfied, the ability to securely challenge previously held ideas and identify significant new information must be developed. LoBiondo-Wood & Haber (1994) extend the impact of reading by suggesting note-taking strategies to emphasize and highlight major themes in gaining initial familiarity with the material. The material should then be revisited, they suggest, and a deeper understanding of the individual themes initially clarified.

Moving forwards in articulating selected research material to address clinical needs requires the structured attributes encapsulated in a planned climate of research-mindedness (Figure 9.1). The characteristics of teamwork are the result of teambuilding to ensure that goals are the function and the purpose of a team is essentially to develop effective strategies to achieve appropriate goals. Responsibility for such action implies critical evaluation of alternative practices. This requires the groundwork of critical thinking and analysis if patient care is to be managed effectively. No doubt there are many more examples of structured resources that can be used to sustain the progress from theory to practice, and this chapter has suggested action research as an additional approach to the utilization and implementation of research.

The intention to improve patient outcomes cannot be left to chance encounters, and the current trend of evidence-based medicine is being matched by the innovation of evidence-based nursing. The Strategic Research Matrix was developed to give some practical perspective to the nurse who feels daunted by the pressure to become research oriented. It offers an accessible starting point which can be implemented at a simple or sophisticated level of research involvement. The continuous nature of the matrix is related to the subsequent production of nursing research, published and disseminated for future utilization. The concept of 'nursing praxis' is ultimately dependent on the integrity of the practice–research–theory loop reflecting theory in action. The author suggests that a day surgery unit could pilot the integration of the Strategic Research Matrix as an element of its management structure, as a means to achieve improved patient outcomes.

DAY SURGERY AND RESEARCH

Day surgery has traditionally been accomplished within a variety of non-residential hospital settings for some considerable time. It was, and is, often termed 'minor surgery' and relegated to the farthest corners of the ward and to the gaps in the operating list. There is evidence to suggest that day surgery has existed, as an established alternative, in Scotland since the 1850s due largely to the inability of the individual to pay for inpatient care. Cost-effectiveness has therefore shadowed day surgery since its inception, and currently the financial consideration still concerns the purchaser-provider dimension. However, its potential benefits of reduced hospitalization, morbidity, costs and waiting-times for an increasing variety and number of procedures, with increased user satisfaction, have been gathering momentum within selective patient-focused, political and professional initiatives. In the relative urgency to sustain and enhance this particular health care delivery system, there is the danger of creating a bureaucratic sorting office, overdependent on the paperchase of guidelines and protocols. Most of these written criteria should contain good research-based evidence, but they do not necessarily guarantee competence when followed rigidly or when they fall foul of incorrect interpretation. Conformity is not an attractive substitute for informed professional judgement and discretion. The challenge to design and implement a sensitive and congruent day surgery initiative that will enable nurses to refine, concentrate and expand the skills that typify it, will need to combine the valid results from a variety of research approaches and methods. The potential practicability of action research may prove to be a useful and expedient option on which nurses in day surgery can cut their research teeth.

The particular content of the chapters within this text, reflecting the sophistication and diversity of skills required in day surgery deserve the focus and attributes of research. It may be useful to the potential researcher or research-user to highlight some of the salient features of day surgery that could provoke thought and motivate action. The seduction may be hard to resist for those who are unaware of the current and potential contribution of nursing, to presume that substantial responsibility for this clinical pathway might be effectively delegated to non-nursing personnel. Criteria for the selection, treatment, care, education and discharge of patients may not be seen to have emerged from, or even be associated with, research that distinguishes the contribution of nursing.

Could there be a research opportunity to establish the particular skills, values and attitudes that distinguish a day surgery nursing 'personality' that confirms the necessity for a professional nursing orientation to promote this specialist form of patient care? Audit, which has strong association with surgical procedures, relates to the outcomes of the practice rather than the underlying nursing structures and processes and may consequently bypass or overlook nursing. Not only can research shape and characterize nursing, it can link with audit to underpin or confirm its authenticity.

There is a remarkable opportunity to research the totality of nursing, in microcosm, as day surgery encompasses the whole patient experience from initial consultation and selection of option, preassessment, treatment, care, health education and promotion, discharge through to continuing care and liaison. Research could place the nurse, consistently, at the centre of the collaboration, communication and coordination needed to safeguard and evolve the effectiveness of day surgery. This attractive option to promote nurse-managed day surgery would complement the consultant-led medical strategies and establish the qualities of multiprofessional teamwork. Day surgery embraces the diverse nursing–medical continuum of patient needs ranging from acute to chronic; trauma and pathology; single to multisystem disorders; recoverable to terminal conditions; paediatric, adult and elderly demands; generic to specialist skills, not to mention everything else in between.

The era of day surgery as a by product of general surgery has been superseded by the development of a speciality in its own right. Day surgery nurses must establish the value of their adapted and expanded skills and roles to reflect an ever-changing focus of accountability.

ACCOUNTABILITY

The commendable initiative of research in nursing has repercussions for professional and personal accountability. The commitment of the nursing profession is inextricably bound to the intrinsic value and benefit it has within society. Research illustrates the very elements that are worthy of scrutiny and wonder, which enable nursing to rely on, and take responsibility for, its knowledge and skills in an informed and justifiable manner. The appraisal of nursing outcomes based on nursing research increases the degree of pride, indeed enjoyment of success, that commits nursing to the pursuit of excellence.

Nursing as a collective and individual endeavour has become increasingly transparent. The explosion of information, disseminated throughout the media, the expectations of today's society mandated within various charters, and the rapidity of change that constantly challenges the status quo, combine to produce an environment that demands attention to accuracy, authenticity and relevance.

Accountability is the endpoint of a cumulative process of gleaning knowledge and taking responsibility for its applied implications. Drawing back from the application of such knowledge does not absolve the practitioner, as the formal nursing codes and the law of the land expect reasonable standards of practice. Nursing is expected to take independent and authoritative action and has little excuse for not keeping its knowledge and skill base current and valid. The expanded and extended roles, especially in relation to the advent of day surgery, cannot rely on the principle of innovation, as it does not reduce liability for any action taken. However, the accountability held by management and educationalists to ensure that enabling resources and skills are made available would complete the collective professional and corporate accountability of a genuinely empowered profession. Empowerment is the process which enables a professional to assert control over the essential factors which affect the means and substance of his/her existence and influence.

Accountability is the obligation to explain and evaluate the implications and outcomes of a decision-making process. It is therefore entirely appropriate that these decisions must be based, as far as possible, on researched evidence. Research in nursing is therefore everyone's responsibility and takes on an ever-increasing role as the catalyst for effective and accountable change.

SUMMARY

In summary, few would dispute the advantages of well-conducted research in nursing and its potential to improve patient outcomes. The esteem and status of the nursing profession is reliant on the quality of its practice.

Research in nursing should act as a motivator to inform and provide the leadership necessary to prompt change. For research to be accepted as an intrinsic part of everyday nursing, it needs to become merged naturally with clinical practice to the point that, without it, nursing would fragment and disintegrate. There are no guaranteed mechanisms to appraise research, and nursing must become self-reliant in its critical selection and implementation.

Research has a distinct role to play, and awareness of some of its barriers and constraints could enable the researcher to discern its potential purpose and options for utilization. The suggested means within the Strategic Research Matrix could generate attitudes and skills that could enable a more productive research environment. Research as a dynamic consequence of human curiosity, aided by the support and freedom to discover, ensures the achievement of the skills that result in professional accountability. No longer should day surgery be regarded as the 'ugly duckling', but, with the advantages of research, it can mature into a self-possessed and refined speciality in its own right.

The impetus for day surgery and the drive towards the positive exploration of medical, technical and pharmaceutical advances is well intentioned. However, its clinical rationale and practice ought only to be considered in the best interests of the patient. Day surgery should not necessarily become the only option for a particular procedure or therapeutic intervention. The future development and reconfiguration of hospital services may emerge from the established success of day surgery as more ambitious procedures require the support of 'hotel' and short stay facilities. Here is the opportunity and challenge for day surgery nurses to conduct and use pioneering research to change the boundaries of patient care for the 21st century.

FURTHER READING

Doheny M O'B, Cook C B, Stopper M C 1997 The discipline of nursing – an introduction, 4th edn. Appleton and Lange, Connecticut
Seedhouse D 1988 Ethics: the heart of health care. Wiley, Chichester
Meleis A I 1991 Theoretical nursing: development and progress, 2nd edn. Lippincott, Philadelphia
Polgar S, Thomas S A 1995 Introduction to research in the health sciences, 3rd edn. Churchill Livingstone, Melbourne
Watson R (ed.) 1995 Accountability in nursing practice. Chapman and Hall, London

---

REFERENCES

Closs S J, Cheater F M 1994 Utilization of nursing research: culture, interest and support. Journal of Advanced Nursing 19: 762–773
Cohen L, Manion L 1985 Research methods in education, 2nd edn. Routledge, London
Deane D, Campbell J 1985 Developing professional effectiveness in nursing. Reston Publishing Company, Reston
English I 1994 Nursing as a research-based profession: 22 years after Briggs. British Journal of Nursing 3(8): 402–405
Greenwood J 1994 Action research: a few details, a caution and something new. Journal of Advanced Nursing 20: 13–18
LoBiondo-Wood G, Haber J 1994 Nursing research – methods, critical appraisal and utilization, 3rd edn. Mosby, St Louis

Mulhall A 1995 Nursing research: what difference does it make? Journal of Advanced Nursing 21: 576–583

Nolan M, Behi R 1995 What is research? Some definitions and dilemmas. British Journal of Nursing 4(2): 111–115

Rolfe G 1996 Closing the theory practice gap – a new paradigm for nursing. Butterworth-Heinemann, Oxford

Rubenfeld M G, Scheffer B K 1995 Critical thinking in nursing: an interactive approach. Lippincott, Philadelphia

Sheehan J 1994 A journal club as a teaching and learning strategy in nurse teacher education. Journal of Advanced Nursing 19: 572–578

Thomson Sir T J 1993 The interface between clinical audit and management. Clinical Resource and Audit Group, The Scottish Office, Edinburgh

Treece E W, Treece J W 1986 Elements of research in nursing, 4th edn. Mosby, St Louis

Webb C 1989 Action research: philosophy, methods and personal experiences. Journal of Advanced Nursing, 14: 403–410

Webb C 1991 Action research. In: Cormack DFS (ed.) The research process in nursing, 2nd edn. Blackwell Scientific, Oxford

Quality assurance

Maggie Fearon

10

■ CONTENTS

CHAPTER OVERVIEW

The promotion of day surgery for eligible patients is based on the belief that a high quality of care can be provided in this way – not just in the pursuit of value for money and economy, important though that is. Quality is a central issue, and patients, providers and purchasers need to be assured that it remains at the heart of day surgery. It is essential to recognize that the patient's experience is the focus of quality assurance.

Day Surgery – A Task Force Report 1993

This chapter examines the way in which quality assurance in health care has grown and influenced day surgery in the UK since the late 1980s. The Government reforms on health are discussed, different models and theories of quality are described, and specific quality issues related to day surgery and examples are detailed. A variety of quality assurance tools and approaches which can be used by the nurse to determine the quality of nursing care in day surgery will also be addressed.

THE CONTEXT OF QUALITY ASSURANCE

Interest in quality assurance in health care has grown during the last decade, and it is now entrenched firmly within health jargon. A great deal has been written about quality assurance in the health service. Organizations responsible for the delivery and procurement of health care have made considerable efforts towards incorporating quality into their agendas. Along with this growing interest in quality, the traditional assumptions of the National Health Service (NHS) have been questioned as the expectations of the consumers of health care have heightened. This has resulted in a change in the organization and delivery of health care in the United Kingdom. There have been many reasons – political, social, and professional – for this interest in quality. The impetus for the quality drive in health care would appear to have evolved from the Government reforms of the NHS in the late 1980s and 1990s.

The NHS is the country's largest employer and is publicly funded. It is not surprising that its expenditure has come under close scrutiny. As scarce resources are allocated, it has become necessary to examine the quality of the service being offered to patients and carers. The Griffiths Report (1983) focused on raising the standard of health care by trying to make the NHS more businesslike, attention being given to quality. This reform increased the emphasis on individual accountability through the introduction of general management and senior directors with responsibility for quality assurance. This review resulted in consumer satisfaction and quality of care being placed firmly on the health care agenda. Consequently, there have been many improvements in service provision and a stronger focus on the patient's perspective. The Government White Paper *Working for Patients* (1989) was intended to improve services to patients. This introduced the main changes in the delivery of health services and altered the balance of power within the NHS. It was responsible for the formal introduction of audit into medicine, nursing, and other professions allied to medicine.

The White Paper saw the separation of purchaser and provider roles, with money following the patient. General Practitioner (GP) fund holders and District Health Authorities (DHAs) emerged as purchasers of health care for the communities served, and NHS Trusts were set up as providers. These changes led to contracts between the parties specifying the level (standard) of service expected for patients. The developing alliance between GPs and DHAs put pressure on providers to improve their performance. Today, penalties in the shape of 'quality bonds' are incurred when providers fail to meet the contract specifications.

Following these reforms, the Audit Commission became responsible for the external audit of the NHS in October 1990. Much of the Commission's audit work is concerned with economy, efficiency and effectiveness in the use of resources. Since its remit extended to health, the Audit Commission has produced many reports with accompanying recommendations. In 1991 the Department of Health issued a Patient's Charter as part of the Government reforms and put the Citizen's Charter into practice in the NHS. The Patient's Charter clarified individual rights to care in the NHS and was launched with the message 'The patient must always come first'. It set targets for service delivery and required health authorities to publish data on performance against these standards. This Charter was subsequently expanded and updated in 1994.

On a European level, there has been impetus for change. Britain is party to the World Health Organization's Target 31, which states that *'by 1990, all member states should have built effective mechanisms for ensuring the quality of patient care within their health care system'*.

The Kings Fund Centre has also been at the forefront of development of quality assurance in health care. It was set up in 1984 with the remit to promote quality assurance in the NHS. It has supported many initiatives and produced several reports in its pursuit of raising quality in health care. More recently it has developed an accreditation system for hospitals to use to demonstrate achievement against pre-set criteria.

In tandem to these political reforms, quality in health care provision was being addressed elsewhere in the United Kingdom. The Royal College of Nursing (RCN) has been leading with quality developments in nursing practice since the late 1970s/early 1980s. The two discussion documents, *Standards of Nursing Care* (1980) and *Towards Standards* (1981), were published by the RCN and reflected the interest in quality assurance. In 1985 the RCN launched the Standards of Care Project and has since produced many booklets to assist practitioners with setting standards of care for specific areas of practice. The standards of care project led to the development of the Dynamic Standard Setting System (DySSSy) which in turn has grown into the Dynamic Quality Improvement Programme (DQI Programme).

Professionally, nursing has become self-regulating since the emergence of the UKCC Code of Professional Practice (1984 and 1992) and the Scope of Professional Practice (1992). The profession has issued its own standards for practice (record keeping and administration of medicines) and for education within PREP (Post Registration Education and Practice). In 1988 an overall plan to introduce quality assurance in nursing and midwifery was conceived. This was followed by the Strategy for Nursing (1991), which made it a target for practice that audit and standards were incorporated into all nursing agendas. Nurse education has also undergone major change over the last decade. The focus of these reforms has been the development of competent practitioners able to deliver high-quality patient care, and education has developed to accommodate this. Many higher and continuing education programmes now incorporate quality assurance into their syllabus.

WHAT IS QUALITY ASSURANCE?

There have been many definitions of quality assurance in health care. Wilson (1987) defined quality assurance as 'everything to do with an organization. All of the pieces of its structure that control and channel life – mission statement, organizational chart, reporting line, job descriptions – set at three of its four corners will be its policy and procedure manuals: administrative, patient care, personnel. And, set at the fourth, whatever passes for an overall theory or model of management'.

Quality assurance is not an 'optional extra' to offer patients and does not exist within a specific department within organizations – it should be part of the culture and daily life of the organization. Wilson sees quality assurance as including performance appraisal and measurement, standards and criteria, nursing audit, norms and peer review. It is clearly about *measurement* and *evaluation*.

■ **BOX 10.1 Donabedian's triad for assessing the quality of health care as applied to day surgery**

- *Structure*: resources available or structure of the service, e.g. adequate facilities, environment, parking, specially trained and skilled nurses and clinicians
- *Process*: the way in which the resources are used such as operational policies, managerial control and responsibilities: e.g. selection processes, written information for patients, pain control, staff attitude, waiting time
- *Outcome*: the results or outcomes of treatment: e.g. emergency treatment following surgery, unplanned readmission, post-operative infection, time off work after surgery, perceived health improvements

Quality assurance is perceived as a way of guaranteeing or assuring a standard of care that is acceptable both to the patient and to nursing. This can be achieved through evaluating both the environment of care and the quality of the care given to patients, and should also include evaluation of the outcome of care. Donabedian (1966) offered a framework to evaluate the quality of medical care (see Box 10.1), in which he described structural variables, the process of care, and reviewing the outcomes of patient care. This is probably one of the most widespread and commonly used approaches to looking at quality in health care today. It is a popular approach used by nursing and has been utilized in the DySSSy developed by the RCN.

Much debate has taken place as to what should be measured in terms of the structure, process, or outcome of health care. The department of Health has set up an Outcomes Group to examine health outcomes. Clearly, within health care, patient outcomes are the most important aspects to measure. It is safe to say that it is not possible to measure the quality of care in a single dimension only, and it is important to recognize the different dimensions of quality, such as those described by Maxwell (1984) (see Box 10.2). This can be illustrated within the day surgery setting, as shown in Table 10.1.

■ **BOX 10.2 Dimensions of health care quality (adapted from Maxwell 1984)**

- access to services
- relevance to need (for the whole community)
- effectiveness (for individual patients)
- equity (fairness)
- social acceptability
- efficiency and economy

Table 10.1 Dimensions of health care qualities within a day surgery setting

Element or quality	Assessment criteria
Access	Parking facilities, ambulance pick up times, ease of access for wheelchair users, waiting times in the unit
Relevance	Determining that the services offered by the day surgery unit are what the population or individual actually needs
Technical effectiveness	Assessing adequacy of equipment and skill of staff, the incidence of complications during procedures and followup problems in the community
Equity	Assessment to ensure that there is a fair share of the service for all the population, and might include analysis of referral patterns and consultant use
Social acceptability	Assessment of the environment of care, privacy, communications between the department and referring bodies, information to the patient, and patient satisfaction surveys
Efficiency and economy	Analysis of 'production costs', e.g. workload and unit cost comparisons with other day surgery units

QUALITY IMPROVEMENT PROGRAMMES

The term 'quality assurance' has been replaced by the phrase 'quality improvement programme', since this reflects the continuous nature and intent of the exercise.

When determining if the service offered to patients is a quality one, it is necessary to measure that which is *provided* against that which is *expected* – by the patient, the community, and the professionals involved.

Quality improvement involves more than just measuring these expectations. It must include taking positive action to correct any identified deficiencies.

When the decision has been made to implement a quality improvement programme, it is recommended that a facilitator be identified. This person should have experience and knowledge of group work and quality improvements and should support the programme through to completion.

Having decided on a quality improvement programme, the first step is to identify the values and philosophy for the clinical area. This may be done by a values clarification exercise, as described by Manley (1992), and should result in a written statement outlining nursing aims, objectives, and values, and should be displayed in the day surgery unit. From this philosophy, standards for patient care, nursing practice, education, equipment, manpower levels and service should develop.

A dynamic, bottom-up approach to quality assurance, involving the practitioners responsible for delivering care, should be adopted, as opposed to a top-down approach guided by management.

Communication is essential in the success of any quality improvement. All group members participating in the exercise should take responsibility for ensuring that the entire ward/unit team – both nursing and multidisciplinary – are kept informed of progress.

Once the standards are agreed and implemented, the next step is to

> A dynamic, bottom-up approach to quality assurance, involving the practitioners responsible for delivering care, should be adopted, as opposed to a top-down approach guided by management.

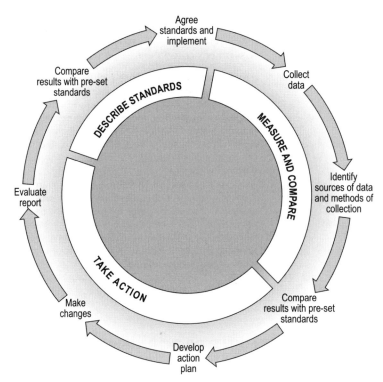

Figure 10.1 The quality improvement cycle. Adapted from RCN DQ1 Programme, 1993, National Institute for Nursing, Oxford.

measure actual practice against these pre-set standards to see whether the service and quality of care given to patients actually meets the expected standards.

Existing, valid quality assurance tools may be chosen to measure practice. Where this is the case, tools should be selected whose underlying values closely match the philosophy of the organization. Following analysis of the findings, an action plan should be developed by the ward team, which should identify the steps to take in order to bring about a change in practice to improve the service. This may involve in-service education or assistance from practice development nurses. Once an action plan has been implemented, this in turn should be evaluated to see whether or not the problem has resolved. This is often done by carrying out a repeat audit of the standard(s). Thus, the quality assurance programme becomes a continuous cycle of quality improvement, as illustrated in Figure 10.1.

QUALITY ASSURANCE ISSUES IN DAY SURGERY

Reports

Different approaches to quality have been described. In examining quality issues in day surgery it is useful to look again at this concept and consider Ovretveit's (1992) three perspectives on quality. He described these as:

- the patient/client's

Table 10.2 Ovretveit's three perspectives of quality in conjunction with Donabedian's criteria

Quality perspective	Structure	Process	Outcome
Client quality: the extent to which end users' satisfaction is achieved	Environment, facilities, parking	Information, pain control, staff attitude, waiting time	Time of bedrest at home postoperatively, time off work, problems, perceived health improvements
Professional quality: the attainment of given clinical and allied care standards	Specially trained nurses with skill and expertise in day surgery	Selection processes, written information for patients	Emergency treatment following surgery, unplanned readmission, postoperative infection
Managerial quality: the efficient use of resources within the limits and objectives set by higher management			

- the professional's
- the manager's.

These can be examined further in day surgery by considering the criteria offered by Donabedian (see Table 10.2). These different perspectives to quality must be recognized at the various levels in day surgery. Quality must be considered not only in terms of the service or product offered to the patient, or the managerial strategies needed to achieve the standards, but also in terms of patient perception and experience. In the pursuit of patient-centred quality assurance, the contribution that the patient has to make in the development of day surgery has been recognized through various reforms and reports over recent years.

The Government reforms on health care brought about the introduction of the Audit Commission. Their first report published for the NHS was that on day surgery: *A Short Cut To Better Services* (1990). The Audit Commission's study focused on the 'basket' of 20 common operations which account for approximately 30% of all surgery. The Commission found that day surgery had not expanded as fast as it might have done, and performance varied considerably between DHAs. The Commission identified the barriers to growth and suggested ways of overcoming them consistent with maintaining and improving standards of patient care, as shown in Table 10.3.

A further report on day surgery was prepared by the NHS Management Executive's Value for Money Unit (1991). The aim of this report was to provide information to clinicians and managers about the management of

Table 10.3 Barriers to growth of day surgery as identified by the Audit Commission (1990)

Barrier	Recommendation
1. Lack of information to measure performance, estimate the potential for more day surgery, and monitor change	Individual procedures should form the basis of performance comparisons at DHA and speciality level. The Commission's 'basket' of 20 procedures should be used to analyse this
2. Lack of appropriate facilities	Specialist day-case units should be provided in all District Health Authorities
3. Staffing	Number of staff per available operating theatre hour, clerical staff be available, nursing staff trained in ward and theatre nursing techniques, rotation of staff as good practice
4. Lack of efficient and effective use of day care units	All cases are treated in facilities with staffing levels sufficient for their needs
5. Improving utilization of day care units	Units should be fully utilized with appropriate cases A written operational policy covering patient selection, information given to patients and monitoring of their satisfaction with the service; systems for patient selection, booking, admission and discharge of patients; arrangements for special groups such as children; job descriptions and job plans, and devolution of the budget as much as possible to the unit
6. Poor management and organization	Proper managerial control should include the day-to-day running of the unit by a senior sister, who reports to a clinical director who in turn has a key role in implementing operational policy. Better management information on staffing levels, utilization of beds and theatres, feedback from GPs and staff. Much more information on the quality of service received by patients and patients' attitudes to and satisfaction with their treatment
7. Clinician's preferences for more traditional approaches	Outcomes of treatment should be assessed by medical audit, good patient selection procedures should be in situ, adequate training in day surgery techniques should be available, the guidance from the Royal College of Surgeons of England on appropriate day case procedures should be updated
8. Disincentives for managers	The NHS Act and Community Care Act 1990 should promote contracting for specific services from providers. Purchasers should be able to influence clinical practices by inclusions in contracts

day surgery and to help overcome obstacles to the development of day surgery. It pointed the way forward in actually implementing the recommendations made by the Audit Commission. The study recommended that, in order for day surgery to be effective and maintain a high quality service, certain prerequisites are considered to be essential:

- capturing the interest and ownership of the concept by surgeons and anaesthetists

- securing participation by a wide range of surgical specialities
- provision of dedicated day surgery facilities primarily for patients who would otherwise need to occupy inpatient beds
- development of agreed clinical protocols for selecting patients suitable for day surgery
- provision of treatment by suitably qualified surgeons and anaesthetists
- provision of an efficient clerical organization for managing the callup of patients.

The Royal College of Surgeons produced a report (1992) which endorsed the issues raised from both these reports. These guidelines also emphasized the importance of regular formal review of the quality of service offered by the unit, including feedback from hospital staff, GPs, community services and patients. This report also called for 'bench marks', describing standard clinical practice in each standard clinical practice speciality area, to be available for all staff.

Patient satisfaction

Since the future development and expansion will be influenced strongly by consumers' attitudes, it has been recognized in several reports that the views of patients and carers and of GPs are crucial. Following from the above-mentioned reports, the Audit Commission of England and Wales asked the Health Services Research Unit of the London School of Hygiene and Tropical Medicine to develop a short questionnaire for assessing patients' experiences of day surgery, one which would be simple to use and useful for clinicians and managers. This was published in 1991 and comprises a single, short questionnaire containing 28 questions (some with multiple parts) covering all relevant aspects of patient experiences. The questions have precoded answers, and it is recommended that the questionnaire should be issued about 3 weeks after surgery. From a sample of 200 it is anticipated that a response rate of at least 65% could be achieved. A computer package was produced to enable local users to process and analyse their survey results. The Health Services Research Unit at the London School of Hygiene and Tropical Medicine has assembled a national database to enable individual users to compare performance ratings. Variant questionnaires are needed for adults and parents of children undergoing treatment.

The field testing of the questionnaire revealed that the vast majority of day-case patients were satisfied with their treatment. The problems listed in Box 10.3 were identified by day-case patients when questioned 1 week after surgery. The Audit Commission recommended that the districts involved in the piloting of the questionnaire should act to improve:

- parking facilities
- facilities for children on wards
- the amount of privacy on the wards
- the provision of (particularly written) information for patients
- postoperative pain control and reduction of the aftereffects of the anaesthetic.

> ■ **BOX 10.3 Day surgery problems highlighted by patients on completion of questionnaire issued 1 week following the procedure**
>
> • *Lack of facilities*: poor levels of privacy, absence of telephones, lack of things to occupy children on the ward, inadequate parking;
> • *Poor information*: in general, short notice of admission or discharge, difficulty finding the ward;
> • *Medical*: poor pain control, after-effects of anaesthetic.

The task force set up by the NHSME (1993) recommended in its report on day surgery that the views of patients should be sought on most aspects of day surgery through patient satisfaction monitoring and that there should be regular consultation with GPs and other health care staff. The task force did not see the necessity for national standards for all aspects of day surgery, but recommended as best practice that locally agreed standards were incorporated into an operational policy for day surgery which set out the agreed philosophy and practice within the unit. This document should be revised annually to take account of the results of audit and the evolution of practice.

The task force produced a 'tool kit' for clinicians, nurses, providers and purchasers to address the particular challenges within their specific responsibilities for day surgery. It contained a number of signposts, checklists and other information on procedures and protocols to enable units to improve the quality of service to patients. It included options for further training for nurses, procedure-specific target setting and purchasing, advice regarding standard setting and auditing, and points to consider when setting up a day surgery unit. The section on consumers' needs included a list of the sort of questions and information a patient might require at various stages of his/her 'journey' from referral to the day of treatment.

The tool kit also asked units to look closely at the following:

• Patient's Charter standards
• issues related to patient dignity
• access to the unit (parking, signposting and access for disabled)
• preoperative and postoperative information for patients and carers
• pain management
• the perceptions and comments of patients.

The task force also suggested some possible performance indicators including: the appropriateness of patient selection, followup arrangements, the proportion of patients who did not attend after being invited for day surgery.

Changes in practice

It is evident from these reports that day surgery units should have examined their own organization, management and practice and taken action in order to meet with the Commission's recommendations for improving standards of patient care. Clearly the recommendations are targeted at different levels within the organization of the day surgery unit and should be acted on appropriately.

The Patient's Charter

The revised Patient's Charter (Department of Health 1995) contains several standards expressed as 'expectations' and 'rights' (see Box 10.4) which should be upheld by health care professionals. Some of these may have already been met in day surgery units, while in other areas action is required to meet these standards.

Professional standards

All nurses working in day surgery are subject to the Professional Standards of the United Kingdom Central Council (UKCC) for Nurses, Midwives, and Health Visitors. These are contained within the Code of Professional Conduct (UKCC 1992) and have been specifically identified within the UKCC's Registrar's Letters and Standards for Practice: Confidentiality (1987), Exercising Accountability (1989), Standards for Records and Record Keeping (1993), and Standards for the Administration of Medicines (1992).

Unquestionably, it is advantageous in day surgery to employ nursing

---

■ **BOX 10.4 The Patient's Charter (1995) – expectations and rights**

Expectations
- staff to wear name badges;
- staff to respect privacy, dignity and religious and cultural beliefs at all times;
- readmittance within 1 month if operation cancelled on day of surgery;
- have a named nurse;
- friends and relatives to be kept informed if you agree;
- single-sex washing and toilet facilities; written explanation of patient's food, nutrition and health policy, catering services and standards;
- clear signposting and enquiry points;
- clean and safe ward environment;
- facilities for safeguarding personal money and belongings; reasonable measures to be taken for your personal protection and safety;
- a decision made about how to meet your needs before discharge.

Rights:
- clear explanations of treatment and risks and alternatives explained to you;
- access to health records;
- complaints investigated and receive a quick, full, written reply from Chief Executive or General Manager;
- advance notification if care is to be given on a mixed-sex ward.

staff with relevant expertise and education to enable the highest standard of care to be delivered. In the 'tool kit', the following activities were identified as those undertaken by nursing staff:

- screening and assisting in the selection of suitable patients for day surgical procedures
- assessing and planning individualized patient care on admission
- caring for patients undergoing all forms of anaesthesia relevant to day surgery
- assessing, planning, documenting and evaluating the nursing care of the patient during the immediate recovery phase
- educating the patient to return home safely to recover in his/her own environment
- evaluating patient outcomes.

Action has resulted in some day surgery units to bring about changes in screening and selection of suitable patients (Reynolds & Morgan 1991); and several audits have been published demonstrating that units are eliciting the views of patients, taking notice and appropriate steps to bring about improvements (Buttery et al 1993).

TOOLS FOR USE IN DAY SURGERY

One quality improvement in day surgery is that of the patient telephone followup survey. This is based on the belief that it is essential to monitor outcome from day surgery to ensure patient comfort, pain relief, and satisfaction.

A great many recommendations have been made in the reports produced for day surgery in the early 1990s, some of which have been implemented and change brought about. One quality improvement in day surgery is that of the patient telephone followup survey. This is based on the belief that it is essential to monitor outcome from day surgery to ensure patient comfort, pain relief, and satisfaction. A standardized questionnaire has been designed to cover all aspects of the patient's experience of surgery, graded on a scale of none, mild, moderate, or severe. Problem areas are identified for action, and patients are asked for their comments or suggestions for improving the care and service they received.

Patient satisfaction surveys are one way of eliciting patients' perceptions and experiences and point to areas for improvement. They do not provide sufficient feedback, however, for professionals and managers as to the quality of service provided in the day care unit. When considering Ovretveit's approach to quality, managers must seek to address many of the recommendations made in these reports, and professionals must also consider their perspective.

Nursing care audit

An audit is a systematic review carried out within an organization to determine whether objectives are being achieved, and whether the organization is effective, efficient, and economic.

An audit is a systematic review of the standard of achievement, which is carried out within the organization to determine whether objectives or goals are being achieved, and whether the organization is effective, efficient, and economic. Utilizing audit within a quality improvement programme can assist practitioners in implementing change in a systematic, bottom-up manner. Audit can assist in the completion of the quality improvement cycle and can keep efforts focused in the ever-turbulent world of health care provision. The NHSME produced a teaching pack for nursing care audit to enable practitioners to develop in this activity in order to meet the targets for practice in the Strategy for Nursing. These are known as the four principles and the eight stages of audit. *The four principles of audit are*:

1. Define objectives.
2. Develop standards.
3. Agree and implement change – then monitor.
4. Communicate to nursing staff, patients, clients and relatives, colleagues in other disciplines, managers and policy makers.

> The NHSME has produced a teaching pack for nursing care audit to enable practitioners to meet the targets for practice in the Strategy for Nursing.

The eight stages of audit are:

1. Gain support and commitment from colleagues.
2. Choose area to audit.
3. Decide who will conduct the audit.
4. Develop standards.
5. Collect data.
6. Monitor and review.
7. Develop action plan.
8. Implement.

Approaches to nursing audit

There are different approaches that may be taken when auditing nursing care. Generic audit tools may be used by practitioners in the pursuit of providing quality care. The use of such tools can enable practitioners to:

- examine their service against tried and tested criteria
- identify strengths and weaknesses in their practice
- identify structural and managerial problems affecting the provision of care
- maximize available time in developing standards of care
- make an action plan to bring about change.

The discussion documents produced by the RCN in the early 1980s attempted to identify the characteristics of high-quality nursing care. It was agreed that both the process and the outcome of nursing care should be considered when identifying good nursing care and that collective professional judgement could be used to determine whether good nursing care had actually taken place. Since good nursing care was defined as being planned, systematic and focused on the individual, it was clear that the quality of nursing care could be evaluated by using the nursing process.

Since then, many tools have been introduced and developed in the UK to evaluate the quality of nursing care in British hospitals. Many of them have been imported from the USA and have been Anglicized for use, while others have been specifically developed for use in the UK.

> Many generic tools are commercially available for the evaluation of nursing care.

Slater nursing competency rating scale The Slater Nursing Competency Scale (Wandelt & Stewart 1975) evaluates the competency of an individual nurse throughout the process of assessment, planning, implementation, and evaluation of care for patients. The performance of the nurse is measured against a given standard, which is within the scale. Data are collected for 6 categories by retrospective rating of care plans and observation of patient care:

- psychosocial and individual components
- psychosocial and group
- physical
- general
- communication
- professional competence.

These are further divided into 84 criteria which are used by the assessors to rate the nurse's behaviour on a scale rating 1–5: rating 1 represents inappropriate action, or failure to carry out action; rating 5 represents best practice. Scores are calculated for each criterion and are totalled, the maximum being 420.

'Qualpacs' The Quality Patient Care Scales ('Qualpacs') was devised in 1974 by Wandelt and Ager in the USA and is a derivation of the Slater Nursing Performance Rating Scale. This quality assurance tool measures the quality of care received by patients from the nursing staff of a ward/unit. It evaluates the process of care as it is being delivered (although it may be used retrospectively) and requires the use of a specially trained observer to perform a concurrent review of direct and indirect interaction of nursing staff and patients. This review includes:

- review of records
- patient interviews
- direct observation of patient behaviours related to predetermined criteria
- staff interviews
- staff observation.

Qualpacs contains a total of 68 criteria, divided into 6 categories:

- psychosocial: individual   (15 items)
- psychosocial: the group   (8 items)
- physical   (15 items)
- general   (15 items)
- communications   (8 items)
- professional implications   (7 items)

For each criterion there is a list of clues to help the observers clarify how it should be interpreted. The patients selected for inclusion in the audit should be representative of those being cared for in the ward/unit, and the ward should be informed and prepared for the audit. The specially trained non-participative nurse assessors observe the care given to a group of patients over a 2 hour period and evaluate the care that the patients receive. Prior to carrying out direct observation, the auditor develops a plan of care for the patients based on the available information. For one aspect of nursing care, it is possible that several criteria within the different categories are observed. The observer rates each criterion on a scale rating of

1–5. A rating of 1 is seen as poorest care; 3, average care; a rating of 5, best care.

At the end of the observation period, the observer collects evidence of indirect care from the patients' charts and records which is scored in the same way. The criteria on the scale are marked 'D' (direct) or 'I' (indirect) to indicate the source of data to use. The level of the nurse interacting with the patient is coded on the recording form. The observer also determines whether there have been any omissions in the patients' care. Scoring takes place off the ward/unit, with mean scores being calculated for each criterion and an overall mean score identified.

Qualpacs has a complicated scoring system and is time consuming, and it has also been suggested that some of the criteria are too Americanized for use in British hospitals, but it has been adjusted in some areas to suit local needs and may be used in the day surgery unit.

Phaneuf The nursing audit by Phaneuf (1976) was one of the earliest quality measurement tools developed in the USA. This is a retrospective appraisal of the nursing process by reviewing the nursing notes. This approach is based on the assumption that all nursing care given to patients has been accurately documented. The audit tool was devised around the seven functions of the nurse:

- implementation of medical orders
- observations of symptoms and reactions
- supervision of patients
- supervision of those participating in care
- reporting and recording care
- implementation of nursing procedures
- promotion of physical and emotional health by direction and teaching.

There are 50 components derived from these functions, which are stated in terms of actions by the nurse in relation to the patient, and in the form of questions to be answered by the auditors as they review the nursing records. It is suggested that approximately five clinically competent nurses (who are committed to clinical nursing, interested in quality control, and able to work as a group) audit up to 10 records monthly, postdischarge, over a 15 minute period. The questions are rated from 1 to 7 for a positive answer, the score being weighted according to the importance of the component concerned. The final score is rated as follows:

- 161–200   excellent
- 121–160   good
- 81–120   incomplete
- 41–80   poor
- 0–40   unsafe.

NATN Theatre Patient Care Quality Assurance Tool This tool was developed by the National Association of Theatre Nurses (NATN) in 1987 to be used by nurses to measure the effectiveness of nursing care given to patients in the operating department. It contains a number of pre-set standards in five sections:

- preparation of personnel: 3 standards, 50 criteria
- preoperative care: 6 standards, 124 criteria
- operating room care: 13 standards, 353 criteria
- recovery room care: 15 standards, 189 criteria
- departmental organization: 3 standards, 77 criteria.

Each standard has a number of pre-set criteria. During the audit, the care given to patients is compared with these and scored appropriately as yes, no, or not applicable. It is intended to provide an annual review of the operating department and should be carried out by two assessors acceptable to the operating staff involved. One of the assessors should be internal and one should be an external person. The NATN have a panel of theatre nurses available to act as external assessors. This tool may be used within the day surgery unit to enable the quality of care and organization to be determined in the different areas.

The generic tools described here may be examined by the nurse in day surgery and discussed with the team. The tools may be used in their entirety or in part, depending on the approach to quality improvement which has been adopted within the day surgery unit. These may both contribute towards and complement a quality improvement strategy.

Monitor and Monitor 2000 The Monitor family of quality assurance tools was developed in the 1980s from the Rush Medicus system in the USA. This programme of research has continued in the UK and now offers quality assurance tools for use in many clinical areas, including accident/ emergency, intensive therapy unit, care of the elderly, paediatrics, midwifery, neurology, nursing homes, district nursing, and psychiatry. More recently, Monitor 2000 has been completed offering a quality assurance programme for use in the 1990s (Fearon & Goldstone 1995). It is designed for use on general hospital wards, but preliminary work has commenced on a similar tool for use specifically in day surgery.

Monitor 2000 provides a series of master checklists of observable quality-related criteria to enable practitioners, who are concerned with the care of patients and their relatives, to set about the quality improvement road. It responds to many of the criticisms of the original Monitor and reflects the more recent changes in professional nursing practice. It embraces the UKCC's Registrar's Letters and Standards for practice, and incorporates the Department of Health directives on discharge planning, the Patient's Charter, and recommendations from the Audit Commission. Several criteria have also been included relating to the nutritional needs of medical and surgical patients arising from the King's Fund Report.

Monitor 2000 contains a ward profile and audits significant aspects of ward management. It also has some 264 criteria which may be put to the patient, the nurse, the records, or to the environment in order to determine a quality index for the ward. The audit tool may be employed in its entirety or may be used to audit particular aspects of nursing care. This may be done with the assistance of quality assurance software programs such as QUASAR or manually at ward level using the text. Correct use of the audit tool involves training and preparing auditors from the clinical areas to ensure reliability, and involvement of ward staff in the preparation and execution of the audit. Monitor 2000 can enable practitioners to examine their practice and make changes in the light of their findings.

Following the completion of data collection, analysis takes place, and the clinical team are given an index of the quality of the nursing care provided to their patients. The results are discussed with the ward team and an action plan developed, addressing the deficiencies in nursing practice which have been identified.

Preliminary work has commenced on developing a Monitor for specific use in the short stay environment of care. It is possible, however, to use Monitor 2000 in the day surgery unit to audit particular aspects of practice, e.g. the named nurse, record keeping, and the nursing process.

Standard setting

The alternative to using a generic, off-the-shelf quality assurance tool is to set standards locally, involving all practitioners from the clinical area. Often standard setting is used in the 'taking action' phase of the quality improvement cycle, in that it enables practitioners to address the areas for improvement in a systematic way.

One approach to standard setting is the Dynamic Standard Setting System (DySSSy). The Standards of Care Project was established in 1980 and has since developed into what is now known as the Dynamic Quality Improvement Programme (DQI). This approach to quality improvement is one of problem solving, and it is based on a number of key beliefs about quality. Quality is believed to be a process of continuous improvement and is an integral part of everybody's work. Collaboration and teamwork are essential features of quality improvements, which can only be achieved through investing in staff responsible for the service delivery and empowering them to take responsibility for solving their own problems at work. The patient is the central focus for the quality improvement process and should benefit from it (Royal College of Nursing DQI Programme 1994).

Getting started

Like any other approach to quality improvements, identifying the standard is the first stage in this programme. A standard 'represents an agreed level of service or performance, and should display a number of features, in that it should be achievable, desirable, and measurable' (DQI Programme 1994).

Writing a standard

This approach upholds the view that standards are written and developed and therefore owned by the practitioners who deliver the service. Where possible this should be carried out with the multidisciplinary team involved in the particular aspect of the service being improved. In day surgery this might involve nurses, medical staff, portering staff, receptionist, medical secretaries, and day surgery patients. It is important that managers of day surgery give support to this system and enable practitioners to take responsibility for problem-solving and decision-making. The starting

The starting point in writing a 'custom-made' standard is for the multidisciplinary team to identify and agree a particular level of service or performance, which is described in the 'standard statement'. The next step is to describe in detail how the standard can be achieved.

Day Surgery Standard

Ref. No:
Author:
Implemented:
Signature of manager:
Client group:

Statement Each patient is assessed by a named nurse within 30 minutes of arrival to the day surgery unit.

STRUCTURE	PROCESS	OUTCOME
S1 named nurse guidelines	P1 A qualified nurse assesses the patient at the preassessment clinic and records this on the nursing record. The nurse explains the role of the named nurse to the patient.	01 The patient states who his/her named nurse is
S2 patient leaflet on named nurse		02 The patient understands the role of the named nurse.
S3 nursing record		
S4 preadmission clinic	P2 The named nurse makes introduction and confirmation within 5 minutes of the patient's arrival to the unit on the day of surgery, and hands the patient a named nurse leaflet. The nurse secures a name card to the patient's trolley/bed; further identification of being the named nurse.	03 The named nurse's name is recorded on the nursing record.
S5 named nurse bed/trolley clips		
	P3 The nurse checks the assessment from the preadmission clinic with the patient and adjusts/makes additions as appropriate.	

Figure 10.2 Representation, in terms of structure, process, and outcome, of a sample standard statement for day surgery.

point is therefore to identify and agree a particular level of service or performance, which is described in the 'standard statement'. The next step is to describe in detail how the standard can be achieved. The DQI programme advocates the approach described by Donabedian (1966), i.e. that of identifying structure, process, and outcome criteria. An example of a standard in day surgery could be as portrayed in Figure 10.2.

Developing an audit tool

Having agreed the standard, the next step is to write an audit tool to find out if the expected standard is being met in practice. This is done by examining each criterion in the standard and identifying how to determine whether it has been achieved. It is important to consider the sample to audit at this stage (see Box 10.5).

> Having agreed the standard, the next step is to write an audit tool to find out if the expected standard is being met in practice.

The DQI Programme recommends that the sample size should be at least 12, and it may be necessary to stratify the sample on occasion into subgroups to capture any differences that may arise, e.g. from variables such as age, sex, ethnic background, length of time in hospital, diagnosis. Thus the audit form for the sample standard shown in Box 10.2 could be as shown in Figure 10.3.

Implementing the standard

In developing an audit tool and a standard it is essential to pilot both, since piloting often picks up omissions or unnecessary criteria within the standard and the audit tool. It also enables the auditor to clarify both the timing and time frame of data collection. Once this is done, it may be necessary to refine the standard or audit tool before proceeding to implementation.

Analysing data and taking action

When data collection is complete the next step is to examine the data. This is done by comparing the responses in the audit form with the expected

---

■ **BOX 10.5 Audit sample considerations.**

Methods of data collection:

- Asking   – patient/carers/nurse
- Observation – environment/patient/nurse
- Reviewing   – records/documentation.

Consider the following in the sample:

- sample size
- random selection
- timing for target group
- time frame to collect data
- who will be the auditors?

Date			
Auditor			
Time frame			
Audit sample			
Audit objective To determine whether the named nurse assesses the patient within 30 minutes of arrival to the day surgery unit			

Target	Method	Code	Question
Environment	Observe	S1	Are there guidelines for implementing the named nurse?
		S2	Is there a named nurse leaflet available?
		S3	Is there a named nurse clip on the patient's trolley/bed?
Records	Review	P1a	Was the patient assessed in the pre-admission clinic?
		P3a	Has the named nurse checked the pre-admission assessment?
		P3b	Has the nurse updated this, if required
		O3	Is the name of the named nurse recorded?
Patient	Ask	P1b	At the pre-admission clinic, did the nurse explain the role of your special (named) nurse
		P2a	Did your special (named) nurse introduce themselves to you today?
		P2b	Was this within 5 minutes of your arrival onto the unit?
		P2c	Was confirmation about being your named nurse given?
		P2d	Were you given a leaflet explaining the role of the named nurse?
		O1	Do you know who your named nurse is?
		O2	Do you understand what your named nurse is responsible for?

Figure 10.3 Audit form for sample standard shown in Figure 10.2.

> When data collection is complete, the responses in the audit form are compared with the expected responses to identify the compliance achieved in practice.

responses. It is then possible to identify the compliance achieved in practice. This then enables the auditor to identify areas where achievement with the standard is good and areas where improvement is necessary. The audit data is summarized and should then be discussed with the team. The group should then interpret the findings and develop an action plan to improve quality. This should include identifying the member of staff responsible for specific action and a time frame in which the improvements should be achieved. A date should also be decided by the group for a re-audit of the standard. Thus the process becomes cyclical.

CONCLUSION

The Audit Commission estimated that, in the future, much of the surgical caseload in hospitals could be treated as day cases. This development focuses on the need to achieve optimal standards of care for day surgery (Reynolds & Morgan 1991). The recommendations made by the various reports described need, clearly, to be put into action if they are to influence and improve patient care and the patient's experience during day surgery. Quality assurance in day surgery should therefore have a predominant position on every nurse's, manager's, and clinician's agenda, and should be a prerequisite in the continual effort to provide patients with a high-quality service in the fast-turnover environment of the day surgery unit. A framework for quality can give direction to the entire multidisciplinary team and ensure that standards of patient care are identified, agreed, and implemented from the bottom up. Careful selection and development of quality assurance tools can enable nurses to measure the quality of nursing care received by the patient and to determine the patient's satisfaction with the service.

Generic quality assurance tools may be used and adopted by nurses, or standards may be generated within the clinical area. Whichever approach to quality improvement is used, acceptability and participation of those involved in the delivery of patient care is crucial. The manager must take action to instil the value that quality of care is paramount. The manager has a responsibility to ensure that quality is entrenched within practice in the day surgery unit. S/he should begin by developing a philosophy of care which should then generate standards for practice. This in turn should then lead to auditing of practice by whichever approach is most appropriate and acceptable to the nursing team. The quality improvement cycle must be completed if nurses are to ensure a service which is acceptable to patients and guarantees high-quality care.

The patient's journey in day surgery is a short one, and every effort must be made to ensure that it is one of such high quality that the patient both experiences and remembers it in a positive manner.

FURTHER READING

Avis M 1994 Choice cuts: an exploratory study of patient's views about participation in decision-making in a day surgery unit. International Journal of Nursing Studies 31(3): 289–298
Campbell D 1993 Talk about teaming up. Nursing standard 7(41): 12–13
Carrington S 1993 Quality assurance in day surgery. The Journal of One-day Surgery 2(3): 15–19
James R 1993 Night and day. Health Service Journal (26 August): 22–24
Moores B, Thompson A 1986 What 1357 hospital inpatients think about aspects of their stay in British acute hospitals. Journal of Advanced Nursing 11: 87–102
Moran S, Kent G 1995 Quality indicators for patient information in short-stay units. Nursing Times 91(4): 37–40
Noon B E, Davero C C 1987 Ambulatory surgery: patient satisfaction in a hospital-based day surgery unit. AORN Journal 46(2): 306–312
Parsley K, Corrigan P 1994 Quality improvement in nursing and healthcare – a practical approach. Chapman and Hall, London
Shaw C 1993 Quality assurance in the United Kingdom: Quality assurance in health care 5(2): 107–118
Sutherland E 1991 Day surgery: all in a day's work. Nursing Times 87(11): 26–30

REFERENCES

Audit Commission 1990 A short cut to better services: day surgery in England and Wales. HMSO, London

Audit Commission 1991 Measuring quality: the patient's view of day surgery. HMSO, London

Buttery Y, Sissons J, Williams K N 1993 Patients' views one week after day surgery with general anaesthesia. The Journal of One-Day Surgery 3(1): 6–8

Department of Health 1995 The Patient's Charter and you. Department of Health, London

Donabedian A 1966 Evaluating the quality of medical care. Millbank Memorial Hospital Fund Quarterly 44(II): 166–206

Fearon M, Goldstone L A 1995 Monitor 2000: an audit of the quality of care for medical and surgical wards. UNN Commercial Enterprises Ltd, Newcastle Upon Tyne

Manley K 1992 Quality assurance. In: Brykczynska G, Jolly M (eds) Nursing care the challenge to change. Edward Arnold, London

Maxwell R 1984 Quality assessment in health. British Medical Journal 288: 1470–1472

National Association of Theatre Nurses 1987 NATN operating theatre patient care quality assurance tool. Published by BUPA Hospitals in London and the NATN

NHSME Value for Money Unit 1991 Day surgery – making it happen. HMSO, London

NHSME 1993 Day surgery: report of the Day Surgery Task Force. BAPS Health Publications Unit, Lancashire

Ovretveit J 1992 Health service quality. Blackwell, London

Phaneuf M C 1976 The nursing audit: self-regulations in nursing practice. Appleton-Century-Crofts, New York

QUASAR (Quality Assurance, Surveys and Reports) 1994 Health International, Cleeve House, Cleeve Drive, Bristol

Reynolds A, Morgan M 1991 Nurses' satisfaction with patient selection and communication in day surgery. The Journal of One-day Surgery 1(2): 10–11

Royal College of Nursing 1994 DySSSy tutorial. RCN DQI Programme, Oxford

Royal College of Surgeons of England 1992 Commission on the Provision of Surgical Services: guidelines for day case surgery

UKCC 1987 Confidentiality. UKCC, London

UKCC 1989 Exercising Accountability. UKCC, London

UKCC 1992 Code of Professional Conduct. UKCC, London

UKCC 1992 Standards for the Administration of Medicines. UKCC, London

UKCC 1993 Standards for Records and Record Keeping. UKCC, London

Wandelt M A, Ager J W 1974 Quality patient care scale. Appleton-Century-Crofts, New York

Wandelt M A, Stewart D S 1975 Slater nursing competency rating scale. Appleton-Century-Crofts, New York

Wilson C 1987 Hospital-wide quality assurance models for implementation and development. W B Saunders, Canada

World Health Organization 1985 Targets for health for all. WHO Regional Office for Europe, Copenhagen

Management in day surgery

Jill Solly

CHAPTER OVERVIEW

This chapter focuses on personnel management and the effect that staff have on the operational management of day surgery units.

Day surgery units (DSUs) may be managed within

- a surgical directorate
- an anaesthetic directorate, or
- their own day surgery directorate.

All DSUs have a common philosophy, whether they are dedicated stand-alone units or day wards with a separate theatre and recovery area; this common philosophy should be the driving force of effective management.

Integration of staff, effective communication, teamwork and good morale is a necessity for patient, user and staff satisfaction.

PERSONNEL

People are our most valuable resource. They must be motivated and used effectively and to their full potential.

A day surgery unit should be led by a consultant clinical director and staffed by a manager, various grades of nurses, administration and clerical staff, operating department assistants (ODAs), and ancillary staff (including nursing assistants, porters, theatre orderlies and housekeepers).

The surgeons, physicians, and anaesthetists operating within the unit should be of consultant status or equivalent and will have operating sessions on a weekly, monthly, or bimonthly basis. These professionals are the day surgery users and are the secondary customers, primary customers being the patients.

Clinical Director

The Clinical Director of a DSU may take overall responsibility for day surgery within the Trust (or hospital), including the budget. The Clinical Director, most frequently, is a consultant surgeon or anaesthetist who is a day surgery enthusiast and is willing to support the unit's operational policies and influence professional colleagues when difficulties arise (NHSME 1991).

The Clinical Director provides support for the Day Surgery Manager and senior nursing staff by acting as a trouble shooter in dealing with problems arising from the unit among the medical staff, e.g.

- inappropriate patient selection
- inappropriate operating list content
- overbooking of operating lists leading to overruns or hospital cancellations
- under utilization of sessions
- late starts and finishes or non-attendance.

The Director's support is essential when increased resources, equipment, space, or staff are being pursued at Board level.

Day Surgery Manager

The Manager is responsible for the day-to-day management of the unit, and frequently comes from a nursing background. The Manager is graded according to the job description and responsibilities. This will depend on:

- the size of the unit and numbers of patients treated
- organization of the unit – i.e. integration with the theatre and recovery and/or ward
- range of facilities and case-types
- number and type of staff to manage
- amount of business management within the job description
- degree of liaison with outside agencies, i.e. NHS purchasers/GPs
- budget responsibility.

Day Surgery Sister/Charge Nurse

The Day Surgery Sister or Charge Nurse has the responsibility for:

- nursing care of all patients referred to the day unit
- discharge planning
- staff management:
  - organizing staff rotation

- promoting teamwork, communication
- sickness
- conflict handling
• availability and maintenance of equipment
• smooth running of operating sessions
• health and safety issues
• training and development of staff, including Individual Performance Review (IPRs)
• maintaining effective relationships with medical staff
• record keeping, to include:
- documentation of patient throughput
- admission/transfer numbers and details.

S/he will also be expected to assist with staff recruitment and selection, and reviewing shift patterns.

Qualified nurses and ODAs

In an integrated unit the qualified nurses and ODAs are expected to work in all areas of day surgery. They therefore need to be 'multiskilled' and flexible to the demands of a day surgery unit. The areas in which they need to be skilled should include:

• preadmission assessment
• ward care, pre- and postoperative
• anaesthetics
• theatre
• recovery.

The term 'multiskilled' is sometimes misinterpreted as implying a Jack of all trades and master of none. If multiskilling is managed sensibly, it is efficient and effective.

Benefits of multiskilling to staff and the unit are:

1. Staff understand and gain experience in all aspects of day surgery.
2. Annual leave and sickness can be covered easily with no effect on DSU activity.
3. Job satisfaction and teamwork are more apparent.

As a result, staff morale is higher, and this is often reflected by a low staff turnover. Naturally, the retention of staff is cost effective.

The disadvantages of multiskilling are:

1. Full competency of all aspects of day surgery care will require a long training period which can lead to frustration of the nursing staff.
2. Demands on the clinicians are greater to support 'on the job' training.

Key benefits to the patient include:

1. Practitioners are knowledgeable.
2. Care may be given by one nurse.

Staff establishment

The numbers and grades will vary depending on the size of the unit, throughput of patients, types of surgery and anaesthesia, and the hours of opening.

The grades of staff and skillmix must match the demands of the unit. There must be adequate numbers of skilled people at all times to deal with fluctuating activity. The recruitment criteria are discussed later in this chapter.

When estimating establishment needs:

- Consider patient numbers, mix, and the special needs of the individual groups. In catering for paediatrics you will need a higher staff ratio and specially trained staff (RSCNs). Lists catering for mentally challenged patients will increase the demand on staff.
- Review facilities and note the areas to be staffed:
  - admissions office
  - preadmission assessment area
  - wards
  - anaesthetic rooms
  - theatres
  - recovery.

Allocation

An example of how nursing allocation can be calculated is given in Box 11.1, and provides a guide to staff requirements.

Senior nursing staff

It is imperative that a senior member of the nursing team coordinates, supervises, and checks standards of care, and communicates at all levels.

Teaching and supervision of students are often provided by senior, more experienced day surgery nursing staff – this should be borne in mind when estimating staff establishment.

Assess the administrative and management tasks the senior sister or charge nurse is expected to carry out. This may include the staff duty rota,

---

■ BOX 11.1 Nurse allocation per shift or per day, depending on shift patterns

- *Preadmission assessment:* 1 per 20 patients (an average preassessment interview takes approximately 20 minutes of nursing time)
- *Wards:* 1 per 7 patients
- *Theatres:* 3 per session or per theatre (allow 5 h nursing time for a 4 h list, including time to set up and close down)
- *Anaesthetics:* 1 per session or per theatre
- *Recovery:* 1 per 2 patients (paediatric 1 per patient)
- *Nurse in charge:* 1 per shift
- *External areas to cover:* as required, e.g. outpatient

allocation of staff, sickness forms, manpower returns, meetings, staff appraisals, checking future booked activity with the admissions staff. A management day each week to complete the administration may be necessary.

Completing a job analysis by nursing grade will highlight time spent on non-nursing duties and will be of assistance when writing the ancillary job descriptions.

Ancillary staff

Some day surgery units have generic housekeeper/orderly posts. Their job includes:

- ward work
- portering
- some domestic duties
- nursing auxiliary duties
- theatre orderly duties.

The average numbers of patients treated daily will allow you to assess the staffing needs for portering and housekeeping:

- Estimate the number of snacks to be made, the number of beds and trolleys to be prepared and made up with clean linen, the number of trips from the ward to the theatre, the number of visits to and from the TSSU department.
- Calculate the approximate length of time each task takes.

There should be a *minimum* of one orderly/housekeeper between two theatres (ideally one in each theatre). This is in addition to the nursing and ODA support in each theatre. The allocation of an orderly/housekeeper to a theatre is necessary to cope with the fast throughput of patients.

Administrative and clerical staff

The importance of having a clerical team dedicated to day surgery cannot be overestimated. They are the key to the successful management of a busy day surgery unit. If day surgery units lack quality clerical support, nursing staff have to put more time and effort into the clerical work. Obviously this results in less time available for direct patient care (NHSME 1991).

Clerical staff are very much part of the day surgery team and should work closely with the consultants and nursing staff in processing the patient admissions. This makes them accountable for the booking of patients and ensuring medical records are available. In well-run units the clerical team are the patients' main point of contact with the hospital (Audit Commission 1990).

The staffing requirements can be assessed by considering:

- the number of patients processed
- the tasks involved in the waiting list management and patient admission process (see Section on session management).

The team of staff should be led by an admissions manager (Higher Clerical Officer salary).

There are many variables when calculating appropriate day surgery staff establishments. The National Association of Theatre Nurses (NATN), the Royal College of Surgeons, and the Royal College of Anaesthetists have produced guidelines to assist with this critical area. However, a regular skillmix review is necessary especially when new activity is being planned.

Recruitment of staff

The requirements to develop a successful multiskilled nursing team are personnel appropriately trained and qualified. Appropriate qualifications include:

- ENB A21/N33   Day Surgery Nursing
- ENB 176/182/183   Theatre Nursing
- ENB 992
- ENB 183   Anaesthetic Nursing
- ENB 998   Teaching and Assessing
- RSCN   Sick Children's Nurse.

There are other useful and relevant courses to consider when recruiting, for example:

- Family Planning
- Computer Skills
- HIV/AIDS
- Counselling
- Gastroenterology
- Management.

Alternatively, staff may need to be seconded to attend courses in these areas.

Multiskilling

Key staff in post should implement and maintain a training programme within the day surgery unit, and develop a tool to assess staff training needs and level of competence. The Bondi assessment tool can be used as a format, amending the contents to suit the appropriate skills and knowledge required to work in any one area.

Assessments for work areas may include:

1. *preadmission assessment:*
   - interpersonal skills – information gaining and giving
   - 'selling' the concept of day surgery
   - health education for patients
   - understanding the role and responsibility of the preadmission assessment nurse;
2. *anaesthetics:*
   - knowledge and principles of anaesthesia
   - knowledge of equipment, e.g. Boyle's machine, breathing circuits
   - paediatric anaesthetics
   - pain relief – techniques and pharmacology
   - knowledge and principles of recovery

- understanding the role and responsibility of the anaesthetic nurse assistant
3. *theatres:*
   - knowledge and principles of asepsis
   - theatre etiquette
   - health and safety, e.g. positioning of patient, use of diathermy
   - instrumentation and maintenance
   - suture types and wound closure
   - role and responsibility of the scrub and circulating nurse.

Producing and implementing assessment tools for each area within day surgery is time consuming. Appropriately qualified staff should be the assessors for the tools to be meaningful, e.g. anaesthetic-trained staff (ENB 183) to assess anaesthesic aspects.

The tool should be used to motivate and guide staff in a development programme.

Shift patterns

The duty rota needs to be planned well in advance to ensure skills and staffing levels match the activity. Shift patterns must reflect activity during the working day and hours of opening.

The Manager and the staff should work together to find the most suitable shift patterns in order to use resources well and prevent wastage. Options may include:

- a 4 day week – working long days
- a 5 day week with some late shifts
- a 75 hour fortnight
   - week 1 a 5 day week (34 h)
   - week 2 a 4 day week (41 h)

Whichever shift patterns are adopted they must accommodate the busiest times, e.g. general anaesthetic work demands more staff than local anaesthetic work.

Patterns will need reviewing regularly as day surgery activity expands.

Effective teamwork

The day surgery team needs to be effective for the patient and for the team members.

Satisfaction does not necessarily lead to productivity, productivity can often lead to satisfaction. The pride and sense of achievement that comes from being a member of an effective group can lead to satisfaction if the individual values the group and the work that it is doing. (Handy 1993)

Handy also noted that the size of the team has conflicting tendencies:

- A large team is more likely to have a greater variety of talents, skills, and knowledge.
- In a large team an individual's talents and skills are more likely to go unnoticed.

The larger the team, the more effort must be made by the manager and senior nursing staff to make it cohesive. If it is cohesive, staff satisfaction will lead to low sickness and good morale. To do this, good communication must occur consistently and in both directions and involve all staff working in the DSU.

Points for good communication:

- early morning team briefings (approximately 15 minutes) to discuss:
  - the day's activity
  - problems from the previous day
  - problems that may be encountered during the day
- a diary of activity with names of allocated staff
- a communications diary for all to contribute (if a member of staff has been absent, there must be some mechanism within the unit by which s/he can catch up with important issues and occurrences, or any changes in practice or policies)
- regular staff meetings (monthly)
- weekly lunchtime debates on relevant topics
- a professional update board placed somewhere prominent, like the rest room
- an information board including arranged social events.

The importance of good communication for patient safety during the course of the working day cannot be stressed enough. For example, the admissions staff, the ward staff, and the theatre staff all work as small teams within a large team. It is therefore easy to separate and reorganize, subject to the demands in each working area. They must coordinate and communicate the care each patient is given throughout the admission to discharge process.

Guidelines for safe practice are available from The Medical Defence Union (MDU) and The National Association of Theatre Nurses.

PHYSICAL RESOURCES

Types of day surgery facilities

Day surgery can be organized and carried out in a number of ways depending on the facilities available:

1. self-contained day surgery unit (admissions office, wards, operating theatres, recovery)
2. dedicated day surgery ward and dedicated operating lists in inpatient theatres
3. dedicated day surgery ward, and no dedicated operating lists in inpatient theatres
4. day surgery beds in inpatient wards, use of main theatres.

The Royal College of Surgeons (1991) says that it is preferable to have a completely self-contained day surgery unit which:

- maximizes patient throughput, keeping the cost per patient down

- provides a better quality service with a much reduced risk of service cancellation.

Options 3 and 4 are more likely to be disrupted by emergency admissions, overflow of inpatient work, and therefore more hospital cancellations.

If day patients are admitted to a general ward, this may cause disruption in an area where the dependency of patients is greater. Within this environment, day surgery patients (fit, well, and of low dependency) may be given low priority. As a result, day surgery patients may be inadequately prepared for surgery and may be discharged lacking the knowledge and information needed to care for themselves at home.

Operational policy

A day surgery unit must have clear objectives and operational policies that reflect them. These should include:

- referral patterns – via outpatient clinic or GP direct access
- patient selection criteria and investigation regimes
- guidelines for appropriate procedures
- timetable of activity by consultant or by anaesthetic types – including allocation of beds
- management of the waiting lists
- booking procedures
- admission procedures, including preoperative assessment
- discharge procedures (performed by nurses in some units)
- transfer to inpatient care
- arrangements for patients with special needs, e.g. children, mentally challenged
- patient information
  - unit specific – where to come and what to bring with them
  - procedure specific – pre- and postoperative care
- monitoring of patient satisfaction
- staffing levels
  - nursing
  - administrative and clerical
  - ancillary
- job descriptions
- staff training and development – rotation through preadmission assessment ward, anaesthetics, theatre, and recovery
- allocated budget
- services, i.e. pharmacy, TSSU, linen.

A separate policy on health and safety is required, which might include the following:

- health and safety audit document
- fire policy (details of fire lectures and drills)
- risk management information (MDU)
- theatre protocols.

The policies should be readily available within the day surgery unit for referral, by all staff and users.

Space

Admissions office

The accommodation needed for administrative and clerical staff must be adequate. In the planning stages sufficient thought must be given to the volume of paperwork generated by such a large throughput of patients. Enough space is required to enable effective management of the admission and waiting list process.

Individual desk space for computer terminals and manual work is a basic necessity. Filing and storage space for medical records is needed. If a waiting list card system is being used, then wall space is required in order to file the cards efficiently and keep them stored in lockable cupboards to maintain confidentiality.

There should be an adequate number of telephones. The number of telephone calls received both from within and outside the hospital is extremely large, and difficulties in accessing the day surgery unit give a poor impression. A direct line is an important consideration, along with fax facilities.

Preadmission assessment

When a patient is assessed preoperatively by the nurse, a room should be available that is comfortable and private.

Staff

Staff changing room space is a physical resource that should allow for some comfort in changing, together with toilet, washing, and other hygienic facilities appropriate to a theatre complex.

SESSION MANAGEMENT

Patient admission process

Once a decision has been made to treat a patient as a day case, the main point of contact for patients should be the day surgery unit. An efficient system for arranging admissions is essential for the efficient and effective management of a day surgery unit. The day surgery unit operational policy should specify who manages waiting lists and patient admissions.

Frequently, day surgery units inherit a patchwork of systems. Letters to patients are sent by a central admissions office, secretaries, appointment clerks, or consultants as well as the day surgery unit (NHSME 1991). This is a recipe for inevitable communication breakdown, both for the patients and the day surgery unit.

The day surgery unit must be responsible for scheduling the operating lists to ensure that:

- there are adequate numbers of beds for booked patients
- there are appropriate staff numbers to care for booked patients
- there is appropriate skillmix for the planned procedures

- the appropriate equipment and instruments are available for performing these procedures.

An example of the waiting list and admission process is shown in Figure 11.1.

Surgeons and anaesthetists who consider doing more day cases, may choose not to because of inadequate or poorly managed day case facilities (NHSME 1991). The day surgery clerical staff will accommodate patients who ring to cancel their appointments, and will find replacements in order to fill the operating list. They will check up on patients who fail to attend, and maintain a valid waiting list.

Hospital notes should be sought in plenty of time so that if notes fail to appear, patients can be cancelled within 2 days of the planned to-come-in (TCI) date. Although this is not ideal, it is a way of dealing with an unfortunately common problem. It does mean the patient is at least given some warning, and a replacement can be found.

Utilization of operating time

Low levels of utilization must be in part due to poor management and organization of the unit, reports the Audit Commission (1990). Delivery of efficient day surgery requires close monitoring of efficiency and utilization of theatre time and space. This means collecting data on patient throughput, theatre utilization, cancellation and did-not-attend (DNA) rates.

Surgical operating time is often scheduled between 0800 and 1800 hours. It is recommended that sessions be planned to start and finish within a scheduled time, e.g. 0830–1230 hours, 1330–1730 hours. The sister in charge is aware of the average duration of common procedures for each surgeon and must have control over the size and content of operating lists in order to reduce the risk of over-runs, subsequent patient cancellations, and underuse.

DSU surgeons and anaesthetists should be of consultant status or equivalent; clinicians have to work within the allotted time, with no margin for error. The potential benefits of day surgery are lost if patients have to be admitted as inpatients at the end of the day, or if patients have to attend Accident and Emergency departments for additional treatment. The Audit Commission (1990) revealed that complication rates together with theatre over-runs are more likely if procedures are performed by unsupervised junior staff.

Theatre utilization percentages are used as efficiency indicators. They measure the percentage used of available theatre time. To calculate the utilization percentage, the following must be considered and defined within the unit, so that staff and users are fully aware and will work together to achieve the highest utilization percentage possible:

1. the start time – the time the first patient is taken into the anaesthetic room; or, the beginning of the first operative procedure (Bevan 1989)
2. the finish time – the time that the last patient left theatre or entered recovery (Bevan 1989).

OUTPATIENT DEPARTMENT

Waiting list card filled in
and sent to day surgery unit

Validate the waiting list every 6 months

DAY SURGERY

Identify a contract
Add to the waiting list

Call patients for preadmission
assessment by letter.
Request medical records

Letters to GPs re 'did not attends' (DNAs)

Give a 'to come in' (TCI) date

Letters to DNAs

Schedule for operation

Record cancellations

Admit and discharge on
hospital information system

Call replacement patients

Return notes/medical records

Delete from the waiting list

Arrange outpatient appointment

Figure 11.1 Waiting list
and admission process.

■ **BOX 11.2 Sample calculation of theatre utilization percentage**

Session time	0830–1230 hours
Hours available	4
Start time	0840 hours
Finish time	1205 hours
Hours used	3.25
% utilized	81

Box 11.2 shows a sample calculation.

Late starts and over-runs affect overall utilization and must be defined:

- a late start – a session commencing 10 or more minutes later than scheduled (Bevan 1989)
- a late finish – a session which finishes 10 or more minutes after the scheduled finish (Bevan 1989).

Reasons for late start must be documented in order to address them, and may include:

- patient's hospital notes not available
- late arrival of surgeon or anaesthetist
- delays to pathology results
- equipment breakdown
- over-run of a morning list
- DSU staff shortage
- patients not ready on the ward.

This way of measuring available and used theatre time, although used nationally, can be misleading. For example: if a surgeon performs four hernia repairs in 4 hours, this may achieve 100% utilization, whereas a surgeon performing six hernias in 3 hours may only achieve 75% utilization, yet the latter is clearly more productive. Therefore, case type, speed of surgeon and number of patients must also be considered.

Cancellations and DNAs

Cancellations. On the day, patient cancellations contribute to inefficient management of sessions. They cause immense dissatisfaction to patients and staff and must be avoided at all costs. Preoperative assessment of patients 2–3 weeks prior to surgery may prevent cancellations on the day.

Reasons for cancellation must be documented and may include the following.

- Patient is unwell on the day.
- Surgical procedure, unexpectedly complicated, leads to running out of theatre time.
- A patient may self-cancel at the last minute.
- Patients may be medically or socially unsuitable for general anaesthetic (this could mean preadmission assessment was inadequate).
- Medical records are missing.

Did-not-attends (DNAs). Patients failing to attend on the day for operation constitute a problem for many day surgery units. It is recommended that if DNA rates are high or start rising, efforts should be made to find out the causes and attempt to reduce them.

Under- and over-runs

Under-runs. If a list finishes early, it may be due to a DNA, a cancellation or insufficient cases booked in. This should be monitored and rectified when putting together the list. An under-run indicates a waste in resources.

Over-runs. If a list over-runs, it may be due to an unforseen clinical complication, a late start, or too many cases booked in. Over-runs increase the risk of cancellation on the day and/or impose extra costs in nursing staff support. If the over-run occurs on a morning list, the knock-on effect means the afternoon list may start late and also over-run. This not only costs more, but has a detrimental effect on the day surgery nursing team, who will be expected to stay on duty. Whilst the staff need to be flexible on many occasions, the morale of the nursing team will fall if lists are consistently allowed to over-run.

Admission rates

Patients who require transfer from day surgery to an inpatient bed for clinical or social reasons, must be recorded by speciality and reason for admission. The Royal College of Surgeons recommends a maximum of a 2% admission rate.

Computer systems

Good information technology is required within a day surgery unit. The software needs to be tailor made for the management of day surgery and should incorporate:

- the management of the waiting list – production of letters to patients and GPs
- theatre scheduling
- production of the operating lists
- the theatre register
- the average duration of procedures
- the length of anaesthetic time
- the average length of stay within day surgery
- late starts – reason for delay
- over-runs
- utilization
- cancellations
- DNAs
- GP summaries.

Many DSUs do not have the required computer software systems in place, resulting in data collections being performed manually, which is obviously time consuming. In considering a computer database, the necessary legal and ethical requirements must be addressed, e.g. the issue of confidentiality and accessibility

Day surgery users committee

It is recommended that a day surgery users committee be set up, chaired by the Clinical Director or a major user of the service. This may prove difficult because of clinicians' varying commitments and may be poorly attended at times. However, the Day Surgery Manager and Clinical Director should encourage attendance and use the meeting for feedback on day surgery activity.

The clinicians have an opportunity to discuss common problems they may have faced and suggest ways to improve the day surgery service.

BUDGET

Day surgery is not a cheaper option than inpatient surgery, but it is preferred by most patients and is better value for money. The economic benefits of day surgery are realized by reducing inpatient bed capacity. Savings can be made depending on the closure of inpatient beds on wards. The running costs per patient (staff and non-staff) are said to reduce as throughput of patients increases.

The opening and operating hours of the DSU must be considered and operational policies written before appropriate budgets can be allocated. The budget allocated to a DSU is often top-sliced from each user speciality budget, depending on service level agreements. Setting a budget for a DSU must involve the transfer of an existing budget to cover day surgery costs.

The highest costs are for staff:

- nursing
- ancillary
- administrative and clerical.

Non-staff costs may include:

- CSSD/MSSE
- drugs and pharmacy service
- linen service
- maintenance (building)
- domestic services
- telephones and stationery
- medical gases
- energy
- rates
- information technology
- catering
- maintenance (equipment)
- pathology services.

A DSU manager in the NHS is usually responsible for CSSD/MSSE, drugs, equipment maintenance and staffing. The remaining budget may be held centrally in the organization. However, Trusts are increasingly devolving more and more budgets to operational managers. If an inpatient operating list is to be transferred to a DSU, the resources must also be transferred.

A DSU will incur the costs for:

- administrative and clerical work
- preoperative assessment
- pre- and postoperative ward nursing
- anaesthetic nursing costs
- theatre nursing costs
- recovery nursing costs
- written discharge information
- GP and community liaison
- drugs
- MSSE and CSSD.

This means a proportion of budget is required from various departments:

- the inpatient ward
- the central admissions office or secretary
- the operating theatre and recovery.

It is advisable to calculate the average cost of a day surgery patient and operating session. The hospital business manager or management accountant should be able to help with this analysis. Medical equipment used repeatedly and frequently depreciates in value and eventually needs replacement – this should be accounted for when setting the budget allocation.

CONTRACTS

In recent years the notion of the patient as a consumer of health care has developed. The Health Service Reforms focus on patients' and GPs' ability to choose when and where to seek hospital treatment.

There is now a distinctive split between purchasers of care (GP fund-holders and commissioners) and providers (NHS Trusts, Directly Managed Units, and private hospitals). Purchasers will only place contracts with those hospitals that meet the needs and preferences of patients.

The activity within a DSU is dependent upon contracts placed by purchasers. The DSU will have contract targets to meet. If more work takes place than is contracted for, activity may have to be reduced to get back to target. If DSU activity is undercontracted, efforts will be made to increase activity.

SUMMARY

The contents of this chapter exemplify the scope of management issues concerned with personnel in a DSU:

- There must be adequate numbers of staff who are appropriately trained who are significantly aware of the day surgery policies.
- They must be skilled in many, if not all, areas of day surgery. The team must be cohesive in order to be effective. There must be clinical leadership to promote and support day surgery developments.
- The administrative team are invaluable and are key to the success of a DSU.
- Good communication between all disciplines is essential.
- The day surgery sessions must be well organized to promote use of the DSU by the patients and clinicians.
- The options for day surgery facilities are variable. Despite this, there should be overall common objectives.
- The budget allocation for day surgery must account for all aspects of patient care.

REFERENCES

Audit Commission 1990 A short cut to better services: day surgery in England and Wales. HMSO, London
Bevan P G 1989 The management and utilisation of operating departments. NHS Management Executive
Handy C 1993 Understanding organisations. Penguin, Harmondsworth
NHS Management Executive 1991 Day surgery – making it happen. HMSO, London

Day surgery as an educational environment

Debbie Hodge

INTRODUCTION

The arrival of day surgery as a key channel of surgical care has had, and will continue to have, a major impact for both patients and staff. Today, with the advances in surgical and anaesthetic techniques and the development of new anaesthetic and pain-relieving drugs, more and more clients are receiving surgical care on a day basis. This new service provides expert surgical intervention for a wide range of procedures in a short space of time. The basket of procedures produced by the Audit Commission exemplifies the wide range of operations undertaken on a day basis.

The benefits of ambulatory or day surgery have been documented (Grainger & Griffiths 1994); for the patient, these include:

- accurate forward planning, with the operations taking place on the scheduled day and at the scheduled time
- less time away from home
- less time away from work
- shorter recovery period.

For the service operators, benefits include:

- fast throughput of patients, making more efficient use of operating time
- easing of pressure on some specialities and reduction in waiting lists
- maintaining high-quality care
- savings on patient hotel costs
- reduction in out-of-hours working.

To meet this increasing demand and the changes in surgical care, the nurse working in this area of practice has had to adapt and develop so that the benefits to patients and to the service operators may be maintained.

Penn (1991) noted that

Nursing skills required for work in the Day Surgery Unit differ from those required for inpatient wards ... different skills are needed where the full spectrum of treatment is compressed into a few hours.

The role of the nurse has changed from one of providing support in the surgical/medical care given, to one of being the instigator in care delivery, for it is the nurse who takes on the responsibility for providing an efficient and precise preprocedure assessment, facilitates correct preparation for that procedure, ensures the smooth running of the unit and, through education and support, empowers the patient to continue his recovery at home.

The day surgery unit provides patients with holistic client-centred care and thus affords to nurses working in that area the opportunity to be part of the whole care episode for that patient. It is therefore a valuable learning resource for the education and training of nurses at many stages through their professional career.

STUDENT NURSES IN DAY SURGERY

Learning opportunities

The learning opportunities afforded in the day surgery unit cover the many and varied aspects of day surgery practice (see Box 12.1). Students who have undertaken Project 2000, degree or diploma pathways may access these opportunities in a variety of ways:

1. during an observational visit
2. during specific rostered and non-rostered practice time
3. as an elective option within their course programme.

Observational visits

For students visiting the unit on an 'observational visit', only some of the seven 'aspects of care' may be addressed or observed. To gain maximum benefit from these visits students must be advised in advance about specific care groups, types of procedures undertaken and the layout of the unit. The careful use of objectives or learning outcomes developed between link teacher and qualified staff, can guide enquiry and provide the student

---

■ BOX 12.1 Aspects of day surgery practice

- communication – interpersonal and extrapersonal, interviewing, patient assessment and evaluation
- preparation and education of the patient for day surgery
- patient safety
  - physical
  - psychological
- anaesthesia
- theatre nursing
- health education and health promotion
- recovery, discharge and followup

with a focus, rather than allowing her to become confused in the whole picture of day surgery. Aspects of care that may provide the student with a 'picture of care in day surgery' could include: preparation and education of the patient for day surgery; patient safety and recovery; discharge and followup. These three areas give the student an overview of the patient's care progression through the unit.

Other areas of care that may provide a valuable focus are:

- the role of the nurse
- care of specific client groups
- unit communication systems
- the workings of the multidisciplinary team.

Not only will students require careful preparation before visiting the unit, but staff on the unit require student information. This should include: who will visit, when and for how long, their stage in their educational programme, what specific aspects of care they would like to access, and who is their personal or link lecturer contact. This information will be required not only for students attending for observational visits but *any* students joining the unit as part of their educational programme.

> Staff on a unit selected for an observational visit by student nurses need to know: who will visit, when and for how long, their stage of their educational programme, what specific aspects of care they would like to access, and who is their personal or link lecturer contact.

Rostered and non-rostered practice

During this stage of the educational programme the students are placed within a specific clinical area to work alongside their clinical facilitator for a period of rostered practice. The students therefore work the same hours as their facilitator and are able to observe and take part in the normal work routine of the unit.

Elective option

In this option, students are able to explore a particular aspect of care in more depth. They, with their personal tutor in conjunction with the clinical area staff, devise learning objectives pertaining to the overall aim of the placement. Areas that may prove useful from a day surgery perspective include: pre-and postoperative pain regimes, education programmes, holistic care, and community followup. Students undertaking this type of placement will probably be in the adult branch of their programme of study.

> Elective options that may prove useful from a day surgery perspective include: pre- and postoperative pain regimes, education programmes, holistic care, and community followup.

Requirements on staff contributing to education of student nurses

A prerequisite for any area taking part in the education of student nurses is the completion of an educational audit. An educational audit provides information on:

- resources
- supervision/mentorship
- clinical environment
- learning opportunities
- staff qualifications
- systems of care delivery.

These are all important aspects of the clinical learning environment. Within this are also the links between the day surgery unit and the college/university staff.

The education of student nurses is a tripartite arrangement between the student, unit staff and university/college lecturers (see Figure 12.1), and these links are vital if student nurses are to gain high-quality education in both clinical and college learning environments.

The link staff from the university must keep abreast of changes in clinical practice and ensure that they do not perpetuate the theory – practice divide. The ward staff need to have an understanding of the students' programme and the part they should play if it is to be fully supportive of the students' educational endeavours.

In order to support trained staff in their role as expert practitioner and student mentor, a number of programmes and courses are now available. One of the key requisites for qualified staff supervising student nurses is the completion of a reorganized teaching and assessing course (in most instances, in England, ENB 998 Teaching and Assessing). This will enable the practitioner to develop facilitation and supervision skills, enhance teacher and assessment skills, and help develop confidence in her role as supervisor or mentor.

An aspect of the role of an assessor is the concept of expertness (Butterworth 1983). In order to be an expert, practitioners need knowledge and skills within their area of specific practice. It has therefore been necessary to provide a mechanism by which day surgery is seen as a specific area of practice and to ensure that, within that specific area of practice, experts are recognized.

The verification of day surgery as a specialist area of care came through the development of postregistration educational courses. These courses

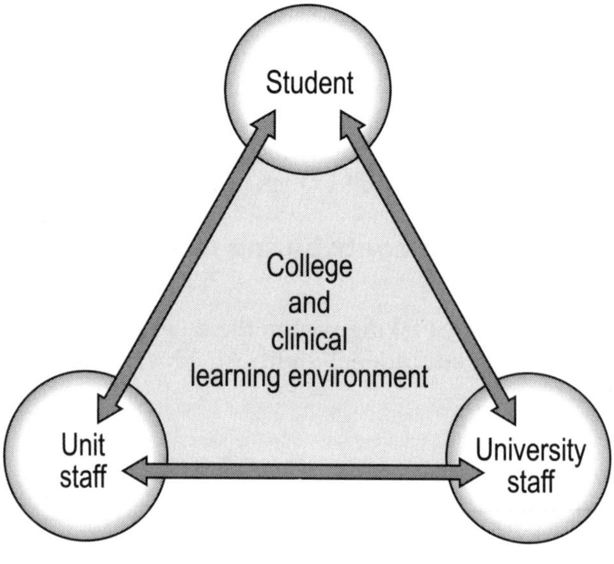

> One of the key requisites for qualified staff supervising student nurses is the completion of a reorganized teaching and assessing course (in most instances, in England, ENB 998 Teaching and Assessing).

Figure 12.1 Tripartite arrangement between student, unit staff and university/college staff.

were formed on the aspects of practice as identified in the day surgery unit (Box 12.1) and the results of a survey into the educational needs of qualified nurses working in day surgery. The survey was conducted at both a local and national level (the latter through the British Association of Day Surgery). The results identified the following areas of knowledge and skill needed:

- assessment, interviewing, counselling
- specific care and discharge planning for all types of patients
- wound care
- management issues
- quality assurance
- patient comfort (pain/nausea/mobilization)
- patient education/teaching
- care of the critically ill patient
- anaesthetic care
- endoscopy
- specialist care in day surgery.

While many of these areas of need could have been met with already established educational programmes, it was felt that some provision incorporating all these elements and linked specifically to care and practice in the day surgery setting would provide a platform for expert development in day surgery practice. A key element of course development was the linkage and interchangeability of theory and practice. This was seen as critical in enabling expert practitioners to develop. The postregistration student is therefore expected to link theory to practice and utilize practice as a validation of theory in all areas of day surgery care.

Another key feature was the concept of the multiskilled practitioner. It was felt that in order to provide a high-quality integrated service, staff should be competent to work in all areas of the day surgery unit: pre-admission assessment, ward, theatre, recovery, discharge and followup.

Courses developed to date validated by the English National Board are:

- ENB A21 Pre-Operative and Day Care Nursing Practice
- ENB N33 Short Course in Peri-operative and Day Care Nursing Practice

and by the National Board for Scotland, P.S. II Module in Same Day Nursing Care. The two English courses meet the needs of two different groups of nurses working within day surgery. The A21 is aimed at practitioners who have been working in day surgery for at least 6 months and who are becoming familiar with the care process and their own role and responsibilities within that care process. The course aims to progress students through competent practice towards proficient or expert practice, based on Benner's (1984) taxonomy of Novice to Expert. This progression is assisted by the linkage of theory to practice in the classroom and by the utilization of theory in practice in the day surgery unit, along with practices validating theory and generating research.

In some higher education institutions the A21 course has been linked to the ENB 998; this provides a combination of qualifications that is needed in the practice setting for the expert assessment and facilitation of other nurses at both pre-and postregistration levels. The course forms either part of Critical Care Schemes (linked with Operating Theatre, Accident and Emergency, Coronary Care, and Intensive Care) as part of an Adult Nursing Pathway and carries specific CATS points related to the host institution. At the University of Hertfordshire the course is linked to the Critical Care Scheme and may be taken as part of a wider degree programme of study.

The ENB N33 is a short course (10 study days, usually spanning 3 months) and, while covering the key aspects of practice, is aimed at practitioners who have spent at least 1 year working in a day surgery setting; thus the content and delivery is aimed at validation and exploration of theory and practice rather than exposition of key knowledge required for practice in day surgery. The course offered at the University of Hertfordshire is geared to meet group needs and reflects specialist practice or areas of need of the group.

The course in Scotland, 'Same Day Nursing Care', has a wider focus than just day surgery, reflecting the specific needs of the nursing population and service delivery in Scotland. It aims nonetheless to enable them to explore the differing issues and areas of care related to day surgery and to equip them with skills and knowledge to meet patient and service needs.

The courses developed to date ensure that nurses have a wide range of skills to enable them to meet the challenges in all areas of day surgery practice, to fulfil the role of a multiskilled practitioner and to be recognized as an expert nurse in an ever-changing area of care.

The continuing education of staff within the DSU will require management commitment in terms of time and money. It will also require a flexible approach to the day-to-day management of the unit if the nurse, having now developed her toolkit of skills and knowledge, is to keep them up to date. This toolkit of skills and knowledge will need augmenting if the quality of service offered is to match patient/client need. The development of the Nurse Practitioner or Clinical Nurse Specialist is the next step. The enhancement and extension of skills into this arena requires imagination and ingenuity, along with a commitment to provide a service that meets client needs (as stated in Code of Conduct (UKCC 1984)).

Four areas have been identified as essential in the development of Clinical Specialists or Nurse Practitioners:

1. skills and knowledge to enhance the development of the clinical nurse in day surgery
2. skills and knowledge to meet the increasing technological and pharmacological advances
3. skills and knowledge in preprocedure assessment screening and preparation and management of that process (including anaesthetic assessment)
4. development of research skills, undertaking research to both guide and validate practice, generate theory and motivate change.

With the development of specialist courses in day surgery nursing it is now possible for practitioners to enhance their knowledge and skills in this specific area of care. However, there are other educational courses that can complement and thus enhance care delivered (see Figure 12.2).

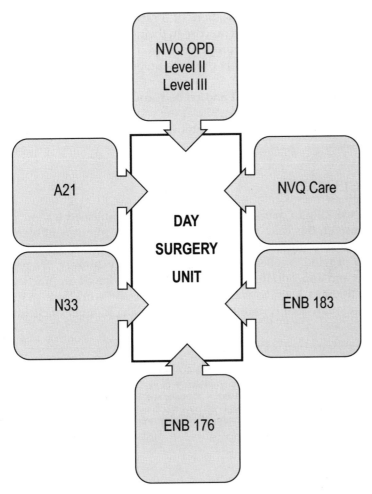

Figure 12.2 Courses or study programmes allied to day surgery.

Through the identification of local needs and skill mix provision, management can, by accessing the variety of courses and study schemes available, create a multiskilled workforce able to respond to the challenges in day surgery nursing.

PROFESSIONAL DEVELOPMENT

Nurses in the UK are now required, when re-registering for practice, to provide proof of professional development and to complete a Notification of Practice Form (PREP Requirement 19).

The key requirements of PREP are:

1. completion of Notification of Practice Form
2. attendance at 5 study days over 3 years
3. compiling and updating a Professional & Personal Profile.

Nurses in the UK are now required, when re-registering for practice, to provide proof of professional development and to complete a Notification of Practice Form.

The completion of a Notification of Practice form is to ensure that practitioners are equipped to practise in their chosen area and are utilizing their qualifications in an appropriate way. This aids the maintenance of a 'live' register of practitioners properly qualified to work in their chosen area of practice.

The careful use of relevant and related study days can enable nurses to fulfil the PREP requirements while at the same time adding to the overall knowledge and skills within the unit, thus contributing to the quality of patient care.

CONCLUSION

Nurses working in day surgery are becoming established leaders in practice; however, this cannot be achieved without a commitment by management to ensure nurses are able to develop the necessary knowledge and skills to provide excellent care in all areas of day surgery. By providing relevant and appropriate academic opportunities based on practice access by practitioners keen to enhance care, an expert workforce may result, providing high-quality care to an ever-increasing number of clients.

REFERENCES

Benner P 1984 From novice to expert. Addison-Wesley
Butterworth T 1993 Clinical supervision. Chapman and Hall, London
Grainger C, Griffiths R 1994 Day surgery – how much is possible. Public Health 108: 257–266
UKCC 1984 Code of professional conduct for nurses, midwives, and health visitors. UKCC, London

Index

About the
PROFESSIONAL DEVELOPMENT RECORD

The United Kingdom Central Council (UKCC) PREP regulations require you to maintain a personal professional portfolio, in which you record evidence of your professional development.

This book provides you with excellent educational material to assist your study and develop your practice. Reading all or parts of it can contribute to your professional development.

The *Professional Development Record* (overleaf) is designed to help you record your study activity in your portfolio and show how it has enhanced your practice. To use the Record, you can do either of the following:

- photocopy the Record and place it directly into your portfolio, or

- use it as a basis for your own individual entry.

The aim of the Record is to help you plan how this book assists your professional development, to the benefit of yourself, your colleagues and your patients/clients.

Further information:

- If you do not have a portfolio and would like to purchase one, please contact your local bookseller or, in case of difficulty, phone our Customer Services Department on 0181 308 5710.

- If you need further information about PREP, you should contact the UKCC on: 0171 333 6550.

PROFESSIONAL DEVELOPMENT RECORD

Book (fill in author, title, year of publication, publisher):

Date of completion of book (or selections from book):

Duration of study time:

Reason for reading the book:

Intended learning outcomes:

Evaluation of material read:

Planned influence on practice:

Evaluation of influence on practice:

Learning outcomes achieved: